April 26,

P9-DNO-876

Hi - Happy Birthday!
Thought you could use
this going into your next
decade. And, the beat
goes on..... .....

xxxx

Spanks x+L

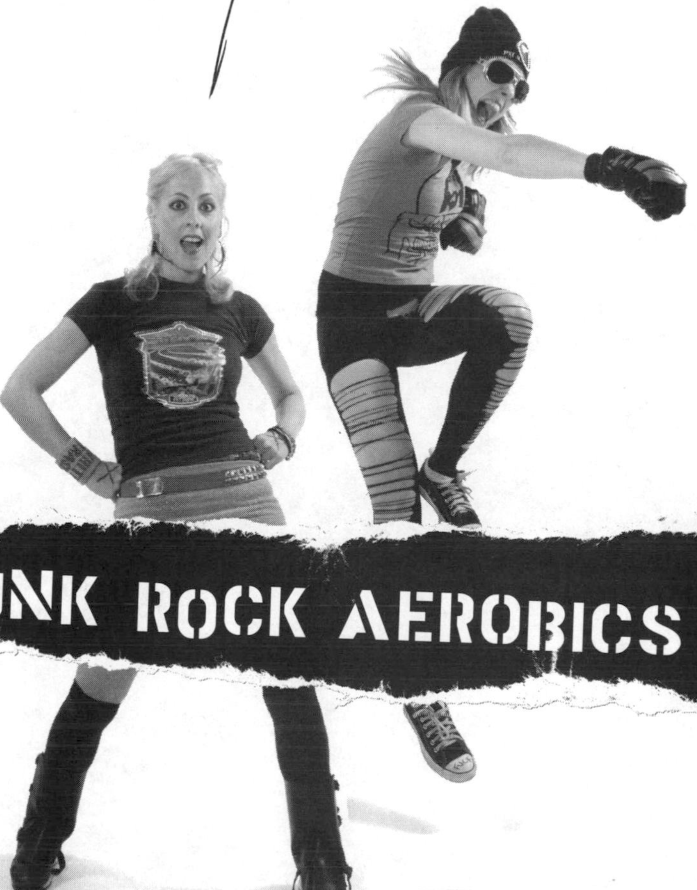

PUNK ROCK AEROBICS

P.S. LOOK FOR DEDICATION ON PAGES 86 + 87

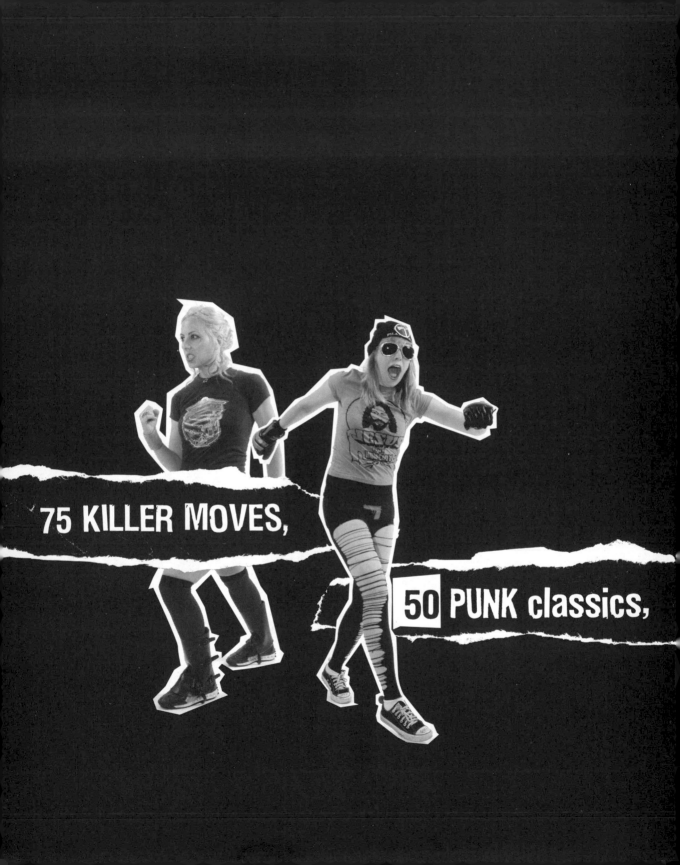

75 KILLER MOVES,

50 PUNK classics,

PUNK ROCK AEROBICS

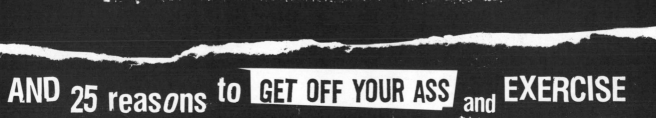

AND 25 reasons to GET OFF YOUR ASS and EXERCISE

MAURA JASPER + HILKEN MANCINI

DA CAPO PRESS
A Member of the Perseus Books Group

Copyright © 2004 by Maura Jasper and Hilken Mancini

No book can substitute for a clinical evaluation. This book is intended only as an informative guide for those wishing to know more about Punk Rock Aerobics. In no way is this book intended to replace the advice given to you by your own physician. The ultimate decision concerning your care should be made between you and your doctor. We strongly urge you to follow his or her advice. The information in this book is general and is offered with no guarantees on the part of the authors or Da Capo Press. The authors and publisher disclaim all liability in connection with the use of this book.

Printed in the United States of America.

Cataloging-in-Publication data for this book is available from the Library of Congress.

First Da Capo Press edition 2004
ISBN 0-306-81339-4

Da Capo Press
A Member of the Perseus Books Group
www.dacapopress.com

Da Capo Press books are available at special discounts for bulk purchases in the U.S. by corporations, institutions, and other organizations. For more information, please contact the Special Markets Department at:

Perseus Books Group
11 Cambridge Center
Cambridge, MA 02142
or call (800) 255-1514 or (617) 252-5298,
or e-mail specialmarkets@perseusbooks.com.

Book design by Alex Camlin
Set in 8.75-point Century Schoolbook
and 9-point Knockout
Photography for all moves by Liz Linder

1 2 3 4 5 6 7 8 9 — 07 06 05 04

WE'D LIKE TO THANK the Commonwealth of Massachusetts for the unemployment checks that helped make Punk Rock Aerobics the limited liability corporation it is today.

CONTENTS

List of Moves   IX

INTRODUCTION: Your Furious Questions   X

1 **READY, STEADY, GO!** Getting Geared Up for Your Workout   1
Rebellious Jukebox   3
Rags, Duds, and Threads   5
Weights, Mats, and Gear   6

2 **DON'T BE A STIFF:** Stretching   9
Warm-Up: Lower Body Stretches   12
Loose: Upper Body Stretches   16
Real-Time Cool: Body Stretches to Slow Down   21
At Loose Ends   25

3 **KICK OUT THE JAMS:** Cardio Moves   29
Basic   31
Footloose   47
Prime Movers   65

4 **RAW POWER:** Strength Training   81
Gettin' Ripped: Arms and Upper Body   84
Never Mind the Buttocks: Ass and Legs   98
Six pack Anyone?: Abs   110

5 **BUST A MOVE:** Combo-Hatching   119

6 **SLAPPIN' IT TOGETHER:** Creating the Perfect Workout   129

7 **KEEP ON KEEPIN' ON**   149
Crash 'n' Burn   150
Big Plans   154
From Apathy to Atrophy   156
Decay   160
Sick of Us?   163
Getting Hooked   165
Last Rites   167

Discography   169

Acknowledgments   174

LIST OF MOVES

STRETCHING

Mono Leg	12
Unnatural Axe	13
Gas Bag	14
Moron Rollup	15
Back Scratcher	16
Cat Scratch Fever	17
Deltoid Void	18
Leaning Tower of Torso	18
Neck Breaka	19
Rock 'n' Roller	20
Ripped T-shirt Stretch	20
Ab Flab	21
Ham Sandwich Stretch	22
Spinal Twist	22
Legs McNeil	23
La Reste	23
Bootlicker	24
I See Spiders	25
Put a Cork in It	26
The Gene Simmons	26

CARDIO

Pogo	32
Skank	34
Rock	35
Wack Jack	36
Cross-Cross	37
Go Go	38
Sideswipe	40
Bacne	41
Circle Jog	42
Dee Dee's Lunge	43
Greased Lightning	44
Ham Curls	46
Teenage Kick	48
Teenage Skank	50
Iggy's Pop	52
Iggy's Punch	53
Thin Thighs	54
Hip Slug	55

Roadrunner	56
Transient Squatter	58
Driscoll	59
Swizzle Swish	60
Swizzle Kicks	61
Rut Dance	62
Thug	64
You Be the Star Air Guitar	66
Super Lunge	68
Roto-Rooter	69
Slits Leg Lifts	70
Head Kicked In	72
Jumpin' Jacked Ups	74
Squatter	76
Plunger	77

STRENGTH

Puss-Ups	85
Biceptual	86
Shoulder-Ups	87
Iron Man	88
The Stinky	89
Chicken Wing 1 & 2	90
Quadruped	93
The Iggy	94
Butterflies 1 & 2	96
Leg Lifters 1, 2, 3, & 4	99
Slut Butt	103
Fire Hydrants	104
Hydrant Plus	105
Face Down Butt Lift	106
Moving Unit	107
Thunder Thighs	108
Scissor Thighs	109
Sid-Ups	111
Meet Your Knee	112
Center Cut	113
Gut Buster	114
Upside-Down Cross	115
Bicycles	116
Water Bottle Torture	117

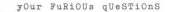

WHAT I
THIS CR

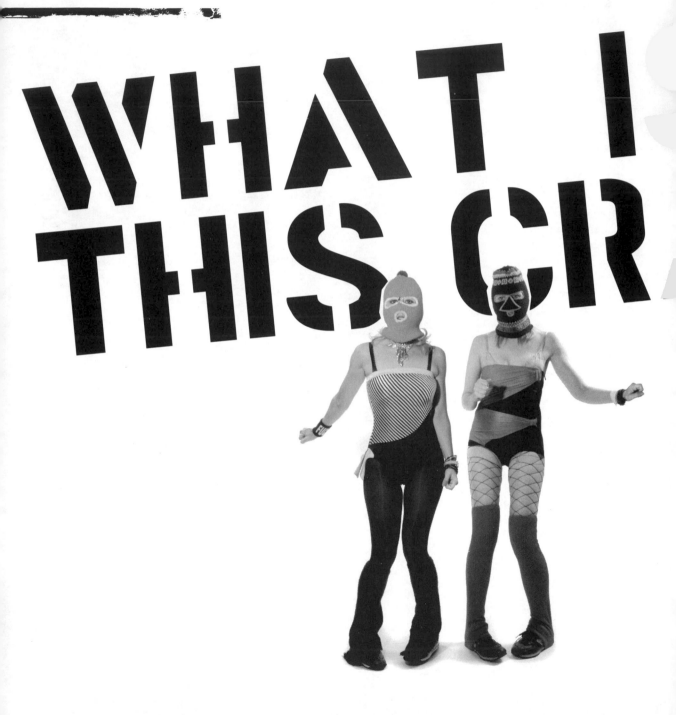

PUNK ROCK AEROBICS—possibly the saddest, most affected phrase you've ever heard. Let's face it, you aren't thinking, "two great tastes that taste great together."

YOU JUST LIKE PUNK ROCK. Or maybe you just like to exercise, but since you've selected this particular book out of all the available fitness manuals, it's probably not aerobics or punk alone that intrigues you. But Punk Rock Aerobics suggests a bizarre union violating the natural and godly order of things: Punk Rock speaks to the nonconformist, the underdog, ugly, unwashed, and unfit. A rejection of the status quo, punk says, "No, I won't do forty side bends to an Alanis Morissette dance remix." Aerobics, though, conjures up images of spandex-clad, squeaky clean, ultrafit Barbie and Ken class leaders shouting through headsets at rooms full of sweaty disciples. Everybody is moving to the same crappy beat, hoping not only to "fit in," but also fit into a pair of pants.

Punk Rock Aerobics is the unlikely combination of punk and fitness born out of a rejection of the conventional workout options. We offer no fitness "regimes" and we mandate no diets. We have no interest in telling you how to live your life, and we certainly don't want you to try to fit into anything. We want to put that "gym bunny" mentality out of your head once and for all. PRA is about getting off your butt, having fun, and feeling good. We want to show you what's cool about fitness and why you shouldn't be intimidated. Getting into better shape doesn't mean that you have to be in a room full of mutants who frighten you or make you feel like a total loser. In fact, it can be easy, fun, and a great outlet for all your angst and frustration at the world.

Punk Rock Aerobics is a totally DIY (do it yourself) workout. Whether you live in a hovel, dorm room, or luxury condo, we'll show you how to get a complete workout simply by throwing some

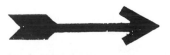

good tunes on the stereo. It requires nothing more than a willingness to try and a sense of humor. Best of all, it was created by a couple of decrepit, lazy, cigarette-smoking, beer-drinking music lovers. Punk Rock Aerobics is for anyone who was ever freaked out by the idea of getting into better shape. This is for those of us who can't afford a gym (and those who wouldn't be caught dead in one). It's for anyone who was ever the last one picked for kickball in grade school or mastered the art of the doctor's note for the Phys. Ed. coach. This is for everyone who loves punk rock music, and especially those of you who operate your stereo with a remote.

WHY AM I READING THIS?

IF SOMEONE had told us three years ago that we would be certified aerobics instructors with our own class and our own book, we would have thrown cans of Schlitz at them. It was all we could do to squeeze into our dresses on New Year's Eve (see below), and we thought that a one-mile walk around the neighborhood pond was an Herculean effort.

WE WANT TO HELP YOU forget about the hell associated with fitness, gyms, and exercising in general. Our inspiration was the scene in Mary Poppins when Mary's trying to get the two little brats to clean up their pigsty of a bedroom. She sings, "To every job that must be done, there is an element of fun … You find the fun, and—" she snaps her fingers, and the clothes and toys fly through the air, whirling their way back into the drawers. The dreadful little children dance with joy, and finally pitch in and clean up, oblivious to the fact that they are doing the very thing they'd been putting off. This is what we hope to do for you. We can't snap our fingers and make you suddenly and painlessly perform fifty leg lifts, but we want to show you how to have fun working at it; exercise is serious stuff, but it doesn't have to suck. Indulge in your own derangement and have some fun—it's time to let your freak flag fly. Don't "stop the insanity." Bring it on full throttle.

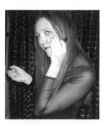

Maura

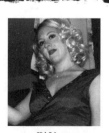

Hilken

In these pages, we will get you set up, get you moving, and show you how to put it all together. We will walk you through everything you need and keep you inspired every step of the way, with fitness tips, cheesy photos, tales of woe, many bad jokes, and reading suggestions for those who want more. There are even demonstrations and tips from real-life rockers who were kind enough to share some of their fitness secrets. In "Ready Steady Go!" we'll help you get geared up for your workout, find the right space, pick out your sneakers, and figure out what you'll need for weights. Once you're set up, you can stop procrastinating and get this amateur hour on the road.

We'll start you off with a series of stretches to get you warmed up before you begin and help you cool down when you're done. We'll also explain why you've got to stretch—but feel free to instead skip the whole section and find out for yourself (the way we did) why you're so stiff afterward, when you can't get out of a chair without resembling a mohawked candidate for the nursing home.

Once you're stretched out, we start cracking the whip. This is where it gets ugly. Are you ready, Cleveland? You'd better be, because there are tons of moves and this is where your heart starts to pump. We will guide you through every strange and thrilling move we choreographed and include some classics we brought back from the dead. Everything from Iggy's Pop to the Teenage Kick will be described in gruesome detail.

Next, we will show you how to use strengthening to build muscle and get rid of all that useless fat. No amount of cardio work alone will get you where you need to be. Weights and resistance work are the key to making visible changes in your body, and if you're as cynical as we were in the beginning, we know that you need to see it to believe it. Weight exercises for your arms, butt, legs, and abs will make your inner Henry Rollins external.

Just as many of the greatest punk songs were written with only three chords (including nearly everything by the Ramones), so too we'll show how you can choose three moves and set them to music. We call this combo-hatching, and you can use it to personalize your workout. Then we'll explain how to build a complete routine incorporating all the elements of stretching, cardio, and strength training—all to fine rock 'n' roll.

In fact, we have the tunes situation covered. We've compiled a discography of more than a hundred songs and albums that we think totally rock. We've also made a list of some of our favorite workout tunes with the time lengths noted so that you can easily pick your songs to make sure your workout is the right length. What do you do if your record collection just doesn't have much punk rock? We made sure to list lots of classic compilations that will provide the Punk 101 curriculum you need to get started.

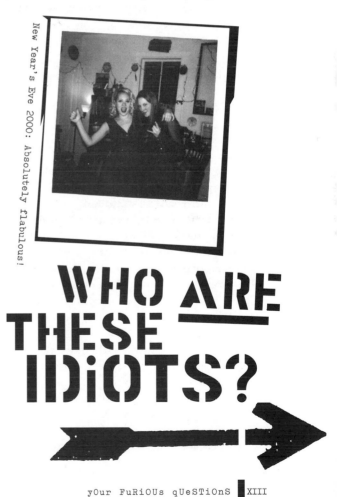

New Year's Eve 2000: Absolutely flabulous!

WHO ARE THESE IDIOTS?

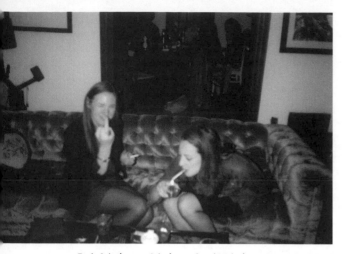

Drinkin', smokin', and sittin' on our butts.

PRA GOT ITS START like most great punk rock bands—with a couple of unemployment checks, a good idea, and a profound lack of expertise. For years, we made jokes about leading an "exercise class" to punk rock music. The concept was tossed around through the haze of our hangovers, when the night before had been spent guzzling beers and listening to old records—suddenly the coffee table would be pushed aside and the dancing would start. Drunk, sweaty, and out of breath, we looked at each other like, "Dude, this should be a real workout ... I'm dying over here!" Losing our jobs helped make it all possible. At the time, we were unlikely tourists in the world of fitness. There we were, Hilken at thirty and Maura at thirty-five, a musician and an artist in varying states of atrophy—two dough balls who'd get winded carrying groceries.

WE BOTH WANTED to get in better shape, but neither of us could deal with any of the things we'd have to do to make that happen. Yoga was hippie dippy, and since we had the flexibility of two-by-fours, pretty tough to stick with. Running required being outdoors, which is not fun during a Boston winter. But these prospects paled before the fluorescent horror of the gym. Not only was it out of the question financially, but a club full of mirrors, crappy music, bad spandex outfits, and people checking each other out under the unforgiving glow of glaring lights was not only spooky, it was downright distasteful.

We wanted getting into shape to be easy, and we wanted to have fun. We wanted to go to a class where we wouldn't feel self-conscious, get hit on, or have to chant or look through our "third eye." We wanted to go to a class free of the trappings of gym culture, where we wouldn't feel we were being held to conventional standards of beauty. We wanted a class where it was cool to wear cheap sneakers and shorts from Goodwill. We wanted a class where it was cool to have zero coordination and no mirrors, so that you didn't have to see yourself leaping around like a goon. What we wanted was to not have to fit in to the established gym culture. Clearly, we were going to have to do it ourselves.

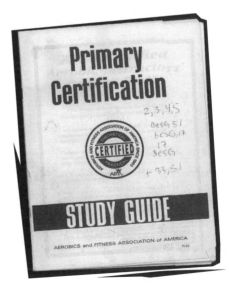

THIS WAS A CASE of history repeating itself. Punk has always been about looking around at the existing options and saying, "No thanks." When punks wanted to see their favorite bands live, they didn't wait around for them to be booked in the local rock 'n' roll venue, where they wouldn't have been able to see them anyway, because they were underage. Punks started their own bands, and when they couldn't get their records pressed by major music companies, they started their own labels.

Starting PRA was not unlike the kid who started a band not knowing how to play guitar. We knew what we wanted—and, more important, what we didn't want. We were also willing to be resourceful with what we had, which wasn't much. Hilken dragged out her Buick-sized plastic wood–paneled television from the Laugh In era, and we nearly burned out its tube forcing ourselves to watch vintage aerobic videos, from Jazzercise to Richard Simmons, turning the volume down and playing our own music while we did the exercises. (You can't properly appreciate Simmons until you've seen him do the Pelvic Squeeze to "Blitzkrieg Bop.")

Clueless doesn't begin to describe our situation. A few things were certain: we would have to train, hit the books, and (worst of all) get certified. Confronted with the dirty business of getting in shape, we took step classes at the YMCA. When Hilken left one session nearly in tears after the instructor ridiculed her for not setting up her step right, we were more determined than ever to bring PRA to the masses. We worked out in the mornings and studied anatomy flashcards at night. At times, it seemed as if we were the victims of some elaborate joke—that we would not only get in shape but would top it off by becoming certified aerobics instructors. We suffered stress fractures and shin splints, and developed a keen fondness for Tiger Balm. But six months later, we were in a crowded gym ready to take our aerobics certification exams.

THE EXAM, OF COURSE, was a taste of hell. The room was full of Jennifer Aniston wannabes, and sprinkled among them were a few who looked as if they lived on a steady diet of steroids and protein bars. Everyone had numbers stuck on their chests. We grabbed ours, stuck them on, and joined the ranks. Feeling like imposters as we demonstrated "rhythmic limbering" and "cool downs" among the sea of gym bunnies, we practically had to hold each other down so that one of us wouldn't flee into the streets of Boston.

The most anxiety-inducing part of the exam came at the end, when we had to lead the group through a floor exercise. Some jocko-dude with a clipboard and a whistle around his neck yelled out our numbers and various muscle groups we had to identify and exercise, "Number twenty-four . . . gluteus maximus!" Despite the stormtrooper tactics, we obeyed. When our numbers were called, we ran like trained monkeys to the front of the class and impersonated normal aerobics instructors. "Hi! I'm Hilken, and I'm gonna show you how to really warm those buns! Yay!" All we ever wanted was to blast the Ramones and pogo. What were we doing here?

A month later, the dreaded letters came in the mail. We waited for one another to get home so that we could open them up and burn them together. But much to our shock, we had become official, certified aerobics instructors.

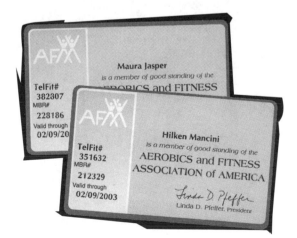

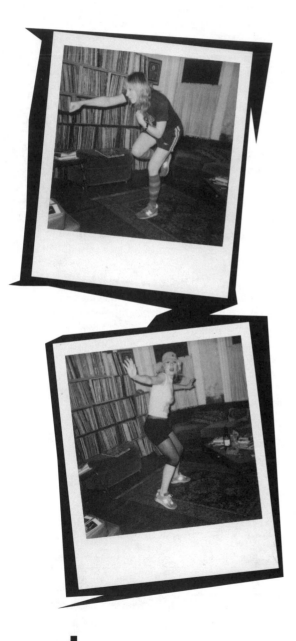

THE NEXT ORDER OF BUSINESS was location scouting. At first, we called some local dance studios, where we were treated like crazy people once we told them what we wanted to do. Then we decided to search alternative venues such as Elks lodges, churches, and community centers, since they often rented out their spaces for "all ages" punk shows. Most of these rentals were found by calling Alcoholics Anonymous and pretending that we wanted to attend meetings in neighborhoods where we wanted to hold a class. We quickly learned to leave out "punk rock" when talking to building managers, but most of the time we couldn't afford to rent the space. Then along came the Middle East Restaurant. As everyone in Boston knows, the Middle East is the home of the local rock scene, and Nabil and Joseph Sater are the mom and pop who watch over it. They offered to let us use the club downstairs on Saturday afternoons, which was big, dark, and had a wood floor. If you could embrace the stench of beer and vomit from the night before (lingering despite the fact that the room was always meticulously mopped before we arrived), it was perfect.

With everything in place to make Punk Rock Aerobics happen, we got to work choreographing moves. We would spend days hanging out and drinking beer; when the coffee table was eventually pushed against the wall, the dancing would start. We knew we could use moves that you'd normally see on a dance floor or in a rock club. Maura would start some crazy jumping move to a Buzzcocks song, and suddenly we had given birth to Whack Jacks (see page 36). If we kept it simple and came up with only three moves for each punk song, we could manage to remember the routine and teach it to people. The motion of the exercises naturally went with the music; it felt like dancing. After the fact, we realized, "Hey! That's just like a punk rock song ... three chords/three moves ... great idea!"

We knew there were people out there like us who'd be stoked to know that they could exercise without joining a gym and acquiring social skills. If they knew that they could show up in a pair of high-tops and cutoffs, bang their heads to the Minutemen, and not get towel-whipped by the popular kids in the locker room afterward, they'd be on cloud nine. So we kept on keepin' on.

After a month, we'd choreographed a good forty-five minutes of music and started formatting the class to have everything we wanted in a good workout. Weights were key, but we didn't think the kind of person who'd be doing PRA already owned them. Since we were still financing this on unemployment checks, keeping it cheap was important. We decided that we could use bricks in lieu of weights, and cheap foam would serve as mats. (For those of you who are poverty-stricken—or just cheapskates—see page 6 for DIY workout ideas.) It hadn't yet dawned on us that we would be lugging these weighty accessories from location to location, but that's another story. We set up a website, plastered flyers all over town, e-mailed everyone we knew, and threw a party to kick it off. In August 2001, we held our first class, and we've been holding them ever since.

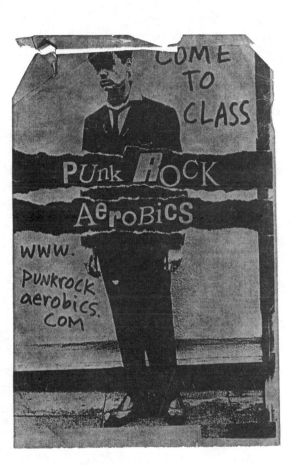

Our early fliers

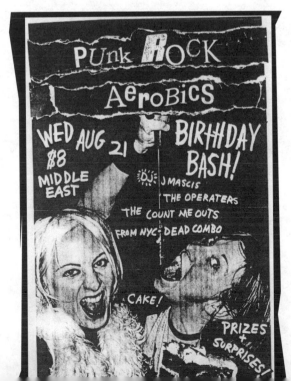

WHEN YOU COME TO A PUNK ROCK AEROBICS CLASS,

THE FIRST THING YOU NOTICE is whatever new CD we're obsessed with this week emanating from a mercifully dark room—usually the dance floor of a rock club. Once you've forked over the seven bucks, you make your way to the bathroom to change and try not to think about what was going on there the night before. If you're really lucky and there's a guest DJ, you might be mortified to find that the musician you worshiped in high school can see what you look like in shorts. But looking around, you realize nobody cares.

There are men, women, and even the occasional little kid. Eventually, we get our asses in gear and get the class rolling with some simple stretches. Before every song, we run through the three moves that go with it, so you don't look like a deer in the headlights when we start barking orders in the middle of the song. Of course, we know you're going to have a hard time and make a hash of it, but our backs are turned, so what do you care? Often, we forget the routine in midstream; there have even been moments when it seems like the class knows it better than we do. We work hard to keep you distracted from your pain, shouting trivia questions and handing out everything from toilet paper to vintage T-shirts as prizes. Once you're limp and drenched in sweat, your masochism is rewarded with a piece of candy on your way out. It's all done in the hope that next week you'll want to come back in. We're always psyched to see the regulars and to watch how some have gotten really good at the routine. One guy's so good (see page 70) and embraced the spirit of PRA with such fervor that we've trained him to teach in our absence. This is what it's about. Anyone can do it, no experience necessary.

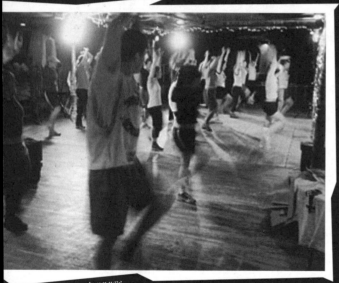

Our class. Awwwww.

Everyone from record geeks to people who have never heard a punk tune in their life comes to Punk Rock Aerobics. There are even people smoking cigarettes before the start of class (and for better or for worse, a lot of them are still suffering from last night's house party). There are teenagers and people old enough to be their parents. Sometimes they ARE their parents.

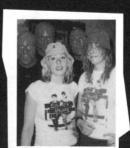

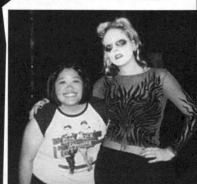

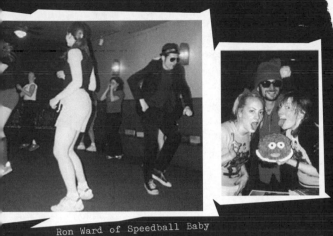

Ron Ward of Speedball Baby

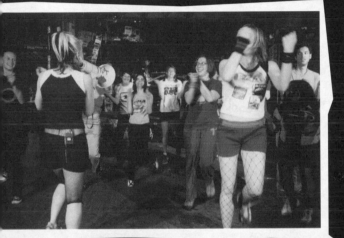

PRA rocks CBGBs

When you come to one of our classes, anything is possible.... At one class, our old friend, J Mascis, front man for Dinosaur, Jr., showed up and played guitar to his song "Freak Scene" while the class worked out to it. He ambled in from out of nowhere and shuffled through the room playing his guitar, oblivious to the twenty sweaty people flailing all around him. Another time, Blue Man Group showed up and worked out beside us before they broke out a George Foreman grill and passed around nearly raw turkey burgers. Evan Dando made a valiant contribution to our publicity by performing our moves on live local television and smashing the station's boom box with a brick. Thanks, Evan.

USELESS INFORMATION

- Did you know that the Minutemen and Black Flag put out an EP together on SST Records called MinuteFlag?

- The Blondie song "In the Flesh" was written for David Johansen of the New York Dolls.

- "For the Love of Ivy" by the Gun Club was inspired by Poison Ivy, guitarist for the Cramps.

- The first Ramones record was made for $6,400.

- Joe Strummer, singer for The Clash, was born John Mellor.

- Poly Styrene, singer for X-Ray Spex, was born Marion Elliot.

- The Adverts song "Gary Gilmore's Eyes" is the story of an eye transplant patient on the receiving end of an executed murderer's eyes.

- Some of Richard Hell's bedtime reading: MALDOROR, by Comte De Lautreamont AGAINST NATURE, by Joris-Karl Huysman

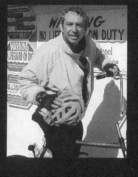

Mike Watt

Punk Rock Hero of the Minutemen

....

Does Mike Watt's cycling regime make you want to go out and buy a bike?

uh, I'm mike watt and I got into pedaling again after 22 years at 16 I got a vw bug and thought bikes were for kids (I was an asshole) and then at 38, this cat in my town here (san pedro, ca) was moving to atlanta and sold me his motobecan ten-speed from the 70s. it's been seven years now and I pedal every morning I can (here mainly when I'm not on tour).

When you think about getting into shape, does it make you think you have to radically change your lifestyle?

well, you have to change your brainstyle, buck the tendency to avoid any physical activity. what helps me is getting right to it in the morning, when I pop awake. that way I don't have to try and talk myself out of it I just do.

Do you have a gym membership?

no. I pedal, paddle, and pluck. no membership needed for a bike, kayak or bass. luckily, I live in a harbor and have great places to pedal along side the ocean besides paddling in the water. san pedro is great that way. I have a practice pad where I work my bass w/my band(s). that gets sweaty too. I do have to pay rent on that pad though.

Have you ever suffered an injury from improper instruction or insufficient knowledge about exercising?

the seat on my bike flared up the place where this illness almost killed me. I got a seat now that only has two pads that hold you where your back pockets are on blue jeans and there's no middle part to f''' w/the johnson or areas near.

Have you ever pushed away the coffee table to dance until all hours of the morning? What songs or records have inspired you to physically move?

john coltrane fills me big time to the brim w/all things wild. it makes me dance in my head.

When you go on the road, do you lose weight or gain weight?

I lose weight cuz the chow is so weak plus my nerves drive me crazy. I get scared before I play and I have gigs every night on my tours no days off. when you're not playin' you're payin'.

Is Frisbee a sport to you or just a major at Hampshire College?

I live in cali and it's definitely a sport here for some for a long time. you east coasters are always late catching up, huh?

Do you like your body, or are you among the ranks of people who think that if they could just lose those ten pounds, they'd be perfect?

I got f'''ed up knees (is this guy a broken record or what?) and funny looking legs. weight gain or loss won't help that. I feel a lot better than I did when I was weighing like thirty or forty more pounds than I do now. it came to a point where I was choking myself out bending over to tie my shoes (my sandbag gut was jamming into my lungs).

As a performer in the public eye, has body image ever been a concern? Have you ever had outside pressure (that is, from a label, etc.) about your weight/shape?

some folks are actually afraid for me weighing less these days. they think it's a sign of being sick. the only pressure I've had is rare peeks into a mirror. also, in the sst records days, my nickname was "bones"—I could eat and drink way more than d. boon and not gain a pound. then at 28, things started to change, metabolism-wise. that illness that almost killed me had me bedridden for like six months and I lost lots there. I also cut out the drinking. I don't know...I don't want to be all vain but I do feel better this way now a days.

Do you think fat people get no respect?

d. boon was heavier man and I loved him tons. people ask me what kind of bass player are you and I tell them I'm d. boon's bass player. he's the reason I play music.

What are your thoughts on Henry Rollins?

I can always count on him, he's been solid for me. he's a strong man.

PUNK ROCK?

THERE HAVE BEEN many heated, boring arguments about how, when, and with whom punk started, and we don't claim to be experts. Was it in the U.K. with the Sex Pistols or in New York City with the Ramones or did it start with Iggy and the Stooges, the MC5, or the Velvet Underground? Although punk seems to have no definitive point of origin, the publicity that surrounded the Sex Pistols added fuel to a fire that exploded with a creative fury and vengeance throughout the U.K. By summer 1977, bands like Siouxsie and the Banshees, the Clash, the Damned, and the Buzzcocks were making waves. From New York, the New York Dolls, the Ramones, Blondie, Television, and Dead Boys led the charge. The music was fast and unrestrained—the sound that fans describe today as classic punk or "old school." The DIY ethos of starting from nothing and playing by your own rules that inspired these bands also fueled numerous independent record labels and fanzines with their unique aesthetics and business tactics, allowing the music to flourish and reach a wide audience.

PUNK MAKES IT POSSIBLE for anyone to be a rock star—you don't have to be able to play guitar or sing to perform. (Have you heard Sid Vicious sing "My Way"? Yikes.) All you need is the nerve to get up and try without caring what anyone thinks. So much about being punk is about taking back control and making your own choices. Being punk doesn't necessarily mean you have to have blue hair, black nail polish, a spiked dog collar, and ripped up clothes. More than a look, punk is about doing something you think is cool, and not giving a rat's ass what anyone thinks.

This is precisely the spirit that gave birth to Punk Rock Aerobics—we had no model, no experience, and it was DIY all the way. When we first started teaching Punk Rock Aerobics, we got countless e-mails from people all over the place telling us that they'd had the same idea; the only difference is that we acted—we got off our asses, and as far as we're concerned, that's punk.

EVERYONE HAS THEIR STORY of how they got into punk. Here are ours:

MAURA's PUNK SToRY

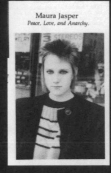

Maura Jasper
Peace, Love, and Anarchy.

Maura's high school yearbook photo, 1983

I FIRST HEARD ABOUT THE SEX PISTOLS in 1977. I was in the sixth grade, and they were all over the news. Some kid clipped an article from the local paper and passed it around the class, causing the teacher to lecture us about what a disgrace they were. At the time, I was a nerdy, nervous, underweight little twerp; my fashion statements were highwaters and eyeglasses that changed tint according to how light or dark the room was. Barry Manilow was my favorite musician, and I'd written him several times to request an autograph. When I first heard of them, the Sex Pistols seemed filthy, vile, and frightening examples of everything evil and bad in the world.

It took another two years for my discomfort as an awkward child to blossom into the full-blown alienation of an insecure teen. I couldn't get a handle on the right clothes, dating, or "making the scene." Gym class was the height of humiliation and I was happy to have a (for me, painless) condition called Osgood Slater's disease, which got me out of gym for a year. Kids were listening to Rod Stewart's "Do You Think I'm Sexy?," disco was everywhere, and lip gloss and Love's Baby Soft were considered must haves if you were a girl.

THEN THERE WAS PUNK. Punk rock looked at the status quo and said "yuck" louder than anything I'd ever heard. For the first time, I didn't care if I fit in—it now occurred to me that I didn't want to. My first album was SINGLES GOING STEADY by the Buzzcocks—I heard it at a friend's house and couldn't wait to get a copy. At home, I scoured my parents' coat pockets for loose change until I got enough to buy more albums: the Undertones, the Clash, Public Image Ltd., the Damned. I started going to shows every chance I got. Most of the time, they were "all ages" shows in the afternoon, sometimes in clubs, but usually in community centers and Elk's lodges. I saw Fear, Mission of Burma, GBH, Dead Kennedys, the Ramones, Bad Brains, X, the Misfits, Black Flag, Flipper, Minor Threat. I shut myself in my room, listening to Vice Squad records and reading zines, and when I emerged, wincing at the sunshine, I sported a buzz cut and ten pounds of black eyeliner.

HiLKEN's PuNK STORY

When I was fourteen, it was 1984, and punk really wasn't happening anymore—but I had no idea that punk was over, and apparently, in the part of Syracuse I grew up in, nobody else did either. My sister had just shaved the right half of her head and was dating the tenth replacement for the drummer in the hardcore band 7 Seconds. People were hanging on to punk by dressing the part and posing in the fashions; my sister was one of them. She ran away from home a lot, so it was easy to go into her bedroom and listen to her records and try on the punk clothes and jewelry that she had left behind. I remember finding a tape in her bedroom that had FEAR scrawled on it and having no idea what it meant. I was a feminine little ballet dancer, but I stole it and listened to it over and over. I was scared by the anger of the people screaming on it, but I liked it, this secret world of punk rock.

THERE WAS A ROCK CLUB called the Lost Horizon at the bottom of a hill not too far from my house. I dressed in my sister's clothes and snuck out of the house one night, paid the five bucks, and got in. I liked the look of the people there: spiky dyed hair, leather jackets with anarchy symbols painted on them, lots of eyeliner. They seemed cool and I wanted to meet them. I didn't think about the fact that I was going to hear live music in front of me—I'm not sure what I expected. The band Die Kruezen was playing—I called them Die Cruisin' and thought that was a cool name. The music was so loud it was painful, and it freaked me out. But I liked seeing all the people who were there. After that night, I went back and saw Lords of the New Church and was afraid of the weird guy writhing on the stage. Later, when I used the bathroom, someone had scrawled Stiv Is Sex on one of the stall doors. Stiv Bators was that guy I had just seen writhing onstage, and I couldn't understand what was so sexy about him.

I went to the club because it was so different, an underworld. The people that went to these shows were really cool, and I liked trying to talk to them. I gradually became friends with a guy in a Damned T-shirt, and went and bought NEAT NEAT NEAT. I befriended a weird, shy guy with a Bauhaus hairdo and an anarchy symbol painted on his jacket, and became best friends with a girl with purple hair in an opera cape. It was exciting. All of my friends in high school were into Phil Collins and Men at Work. I began to associate being cool with going out and seeing loud music I had never heard of and wasn't popular. It was entering into a world that I never knew existed, and all I really cared about—more than the music—were the friends I was making.

I got a job at a record store and decided to wear all black. Not surprisingly, I constantly listened to the Cure. I suddenly did not give a shit if I was pretty or popular in high school. I quit my ballet lessons. I could stop trying to make people like me and just be myself. Even though I made my hair silver and secretly wanted to be in a rock band and write songs, somehow this punk thing seemed not for me, it was more my sister's thing. I cared more about the fact that I had made some really cool friends, and stopped trying to be punk. Later on, I realized what a huge poseur I was, and that I really didn't know anything about punk rock. But the small taste of punk I experienced early on showed me that it was okay not to be like everyone else. I met people who wanted to write poetry or travel in Europe or write songs or plays or join bands and tour—not get normal day jobs. All those people I befriended were punk in their own way, and punk showed me I could be my own kind of freak.

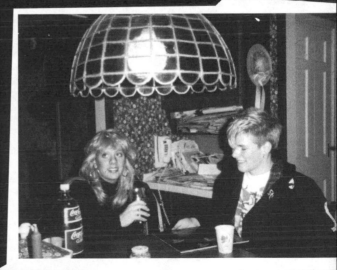

Hilken with friend, 1987

STIV IS SEX

PUNK ROCK BOOKS WE LOVE

ENGLAND'S DREAMING, by Jon Savage. The King James Bible of U.K. punk. A tome of Pulitzer-worthy reporting and analysis, topped off with a Kaballah-length discography.

PLEASE KILL ME: THE UNCENSORED ORAL HISTORY OF PUNK ROCK, by Legs McNeil. Written by the man who claims to have invented the term Punk, this book provides a complete oral history of the punk scene in New York City in the heyday of CBGBs, featuring Johnny Thunders, Patti Smith, Dee Dee Ramone, and anyone else you can think of who was there.

AMERICAN HARDCORE: A TRIBAL HISTORY, by Steven Blush. Find out more about the different scenes and bands that formed the backbone of American hardcore in the early eighties. If you like Black Flag, Dead Kennedys, Bad Brains, and Minor Threat, you might actually start spending nights at home in an armchair if you buy this book. It's full of great interviews, photos, and flyers.

THE PHILOSOPHY OF PUNK: MORE THAN NOISE, by Craig O'Hara. Punk rock as an attitude and a way of life. This book takes a stab at punk rock as a movement with significant political and social implications, and is particularly thorough on the concept of DIY. In fact, O'Hara initially "published" it himself, via Kinko's.

PUNK DIARY 1970–1979, by George Gimarc. The first time we opened this book, the print was so small and there were so many facts and names that we thought we were reading a Manhattan phone book. If you're looking for colorful stories and poetic descriptions, this is not the book for you. If getting the facts (and they are all here) in chronological order is your bag, grab this one. It could easily be the most definitive reference book on punk rock. If you give it a chance you'll be blown away by the accuracy and detail, and, much to your surprise, hopelessly sucked in.

ROTTEN: NO IRISH, NO BLACKS, NO DOGS, by Johnny Lydon. Johnny Rotten's autobiography recounts his childhood as the working-class son of Irish immigrants and the rise and fall of the Sex Pistols. It's strong on stories about the U.K. punk scene before everything exploded. Did you know that Lydon dated and eventually married the mother of the Slits' Ari Up?

OUR BAND COULD BE YOUR LIFE: SCENES FROM THE AMERICAN INDIE UNDERGROUND 1981–1991, by Michael Azerrad. An impeccably researched book that hashes out how some of the most influential bands of the American post-punk indie scene got their start and made their mark. Covers the Minutemen, Dinosaur Jr., Sonic Youth, Butthole Surfers, and many more.

I NEED MORE, by Iggy Pop. Tales from a rebellious adolescence in Ann Arbor, Michigan, and an even more rebellious trek into adulthood. Essential reading if you love The Stooges.

MAKING TRACKS: THE RISE OF BLONDIE, by Debbie Harry, Chris Stein, and Victor Bockris. Reading this book makes any episode of Behind the Music look like a tawdry success story. Making Tracks is an honest and candid tale of struggle with an extra helping of photos of its photogenic heroine. It's also refreshingly humble, and makes you feel that success wasn't wasted on this band.

AND I DON'T WANNA LIVE THIS LIFE, by Deborah Spungen. The story of Nancy Spungen, main squeeze of Sid Vicious, told through the eyes of her mother. The Mommie Dearest of punk rock—only intended to be more like Daughter Dearest. It whets your appetite for the Courtney Love story as told by her dad; if only her lawyers would let it happen.

AEROBICS?

NOW THAT YOU'VE WISED UP to punk, it's time to get hip to exercise. Any moron knows that exercise is good for you. We wish we could tell you ignorance is bliss, teach you a few moves, and call it a day. But somehow, just getting the information about exercise is never enough to motivate someone to start working out and stay at it. Most people are excellent at denial. Does anyone really care what the Surgeon General has to say about cigarettes and booze? It's hard to avoid the onslaught of health information currently available. Health breakthroughs and studies are headline news, and even the dumbest fashion magazines and tabloids tell you how to count calories and rid yourself of Bingo Arm (see page 90). For a lot of us, though, it's in one ear and out the other—or, to cop a phrase from Minor Threat, "It's like screamin' at a wall."

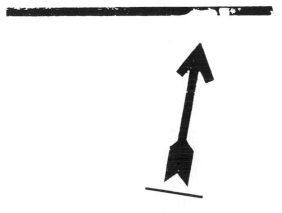

IT'S EASY TO IGNORE THE FACTS, because sometimes the bad stuff is really satisfying—once you've started on a bag of Lays and you're halfway through another episode of Golddiggers' Tropical Millionaire Search, chances are you feel happy as a clam. It's easy to succumb to the rewards of immediate gratification—especially if it's all you know. In the same way that smokers don't know how good it feels not to smoke, it's nearly impossible to convey how good exercise will make you feel both immediately and in the long term. The first ten minutes of working out can feel like running through a bog. But stick it out and you'll feel invigorated, relaxed, and possibly even proud that you actually did it. (There's more on your excuses—we've heard 'em all—our encouragement, and why you ought to shut up and put up on page 157.)

But if you make it through the first ten minutes of one of our workouts and can keep going for at least twenty-five, here are some of the good things you can expect, right away. First, you should be sweating like a pig, or at least have broken a sweat. When you sweat, toxins are released and eliminated through the pores of your skin; it's one of the best ways to detox from last night's party. In addition, your heart and lungs will also be working harder to pump blood more efficiently throughout your body. This brings a greater supply of oxygen to your brain and just about everywhere else. You'll have a healthy glow and feel much more alert.

If you're nervous or suffer from anxiety, exercise will take the edge off so that you won't drive people nuts with your incessant air drumming and foot tapping. If you are really lucky, you might even get the endorphin rush known as runner's high.

When you're done working out, your metabolism will be racing, so feel free to attack that slice of pizza, and know that when it's time to pass out, you're probably going to have a much sounder sleep. Visions of fairies and unicorns might inhabit your dreams, replacing the usual alien abduction.

If you can really commit to regular exercise, the benefits are overwhelming.

- You'll build a stronger heart that pumps more oxygenated blood without having to work as hard. That lessens your chance of having a heart attack in the middle of a stage dive or a pogo frenzy in your living room.

- Exercise increases the number and size of blood vessels, which both lowers blood pressure and increases lung capacity. So even if you haven't kicked your pack-a-day habit, at least you're breathing better and getting more oxygen in your body.

- Exercise will make you stronger—you'll replace fat with firm muscle. If you need to kick someone's ass, there's some possibility you'll succeed.

ENDORPHINS ARE CHEMICALS released by your pituitary gland after prolonged periods of physical stress, pain, and sometimes exercise. They function as "natural painkillers" and have been known to make people feel euphoric.

- Exercise builds greater bone density, greatly lowering your risk of developing osteoporosis, the disease that will crumble your bones and make you shrink as you age.

- Exercise will improve your posture, helping to straighten your back and open your shoulders so that you can finally stop slouching like the living dead.

- Exercise will improve your balance and coordination and increase your range of motion, so when you want to kick out the jams on the dance floor, you won't move like our slothlike friend, J Mascis.

- Exercise will give you increased endurance, so once you've stolen the dance floor and closed the bar, you can head off to that after-hours party, where you'll realize that you are the only person not high on booger sugar.

- Exercise builds resistance to illness and lowers your risk of getting cancer, having a stroke, and developing adult onset diabetes.

It's so good, it almost sounds like a scam ... and that's only half the story.

NOT ONLY DO YOU feel good about taking control; it feels great when you actually see your body start to change and grow little muscles. Studies have linked exercise to overall improvements in mood, a reduction in stress and anxiety, and relief from symptoms of depression. Such a pursuit of happiness might sound conformist and lame to some—but is upping the Zoloft prescription a better idea? Some people claim that exercise has even helped improve their social skills and sex lives. So you can say good-bye to hours sulking in your room to Joy Division and the Smiths. (If you choose to cut down on Joy Division time, that is; we're the last ones to tell you to stop listening to records and get some sunshine.) Regular aerobic activity has been proven to improve memory and also to offset age-related dementia.

Here's the holier-than-thou, gloom-and-doom part:

- By not exercising, you put yourself more at risk for developing a host of age- and neglect-related diseases.

- Your body will start to rot like a car in a junk heap, turning you into an atrophied blob with brittle bones.

- You will get run over pushing a cart at the supermarket, and even the clapper won't be able to save you.

- You will be more prone to developing arthritis, diabetes, poor circulation, heart disease, depression, obesity, loss of self-esteem, lethargy, osteoporosis, weakened immune system, premature aging, and social isolation (since you won't be able to do too much).

The list goes on. It'll be all you can do to get out of bed and limp to your dumb job or practice space in the morning. That's not punk rock.

Kathy Foster
the Thermals

What are your thoughts on Danzig?

Short and Buff.

Does Richard Simmons make you laugh or make you think of a scary clown?

That guy is OOC! (out of control)

When you think about getting into shape, does it make you think you have to radically change your lifestyle?

Kinda. I'd have to make time, get up ... y'know. It would really cut into my TV and drug time.

If you exercise, what type of exercise do you do? And what kind of music do you listen to when working out?

I like to swim, silently, and dance to lots of stuff —James Brown, Ramones, Flaming Lips, Le Tigre, whatever, the Friends theme song but I hate f---in 80s night. Lame!

Have you ever pushed away the coffee table to dance until all hours of the morning?

Coffee table? Morning?

If you're on the road and one of your bandmates or fellow touring bands gets up to go for a jog, do you hate them or join them?

Ha ha ha ha ha ha ha ... ohhhhhh, good one!

Do you like your body, or are you among the ranks of people who think that if they could just lose those ten pounds, they'd be perfect?

My bod is the s--t. I mean, look at me!

As a performer in the public eye, has body image ever been a concern? Have you ever had outside pressure (that is, from a label, etc.) about your weight/shape?

Nah, I'm more concerned with whether my hair is stringy and messed-up-looking enough, and if my jeans are cool and my converse aren't too new-looking, and whether my army surplus looks surplussy enough. Oh wait, I'm not in the Strokes. Nevermind.

Are you afraid of dodgeball?

Bring it.

P.R.A. Q&A #2

Britta Phillips

Bass Player for Luna

....

Does Mike Watt's cycling regimen make you want to go out and buy a bike?

No. I didn't know about his cycling regime, but I think a bike's a pain in the ass in New York City.

If you exercise, what type of exercise do you do? And what kind of music do you listen to when you work out?

These days I run on the treadmill at the gym. My current music mix includes The Stooges, New Order, Lou Reed, The Velvet Underground, The Stones, Voidoids, Talking Heads, Them, Ladytron, Clinic and Spacemen 3.

Does Natalie Merchant's interpretive dancing inspire you?

Blech!

If you're on the road and one of your bandmates or fellow touring bands gets up to go for a jog, do you hate them or join them?

That depends on how late I stayed up the night before … if I've been "good," then I'd probably like to join them.

Has your state of "being in shape" ever affected your performance either positively or negatively? Do you tend to work up a sweat onstage?

Sometimes I sweat onstage, but that's usually due to the club climate not because I move around that much. I do think I get tired out too quickly if I haven't been exercising, though. And I feel more confident and aggressive if I'm in shape.

As a performer in the public eye, has body image ever been a concern? Have you ever had outside pressure (that is, from a label, etc.) about your weight/shape?

Of course. I've never gotten any external pressure (although everyone always cheers weight loss) but I've certainly felt my own internal pressure which has been influenced by the entertainment media's impossible standards.

Is skinny better than buff?

No. To be healthy and feel good, you gotta get a little muscle tone. But there are different body types and some people are naturally thinner or more muscular, or rounder and softer.

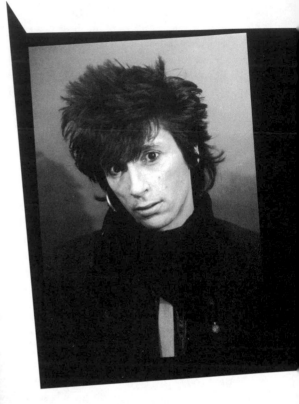

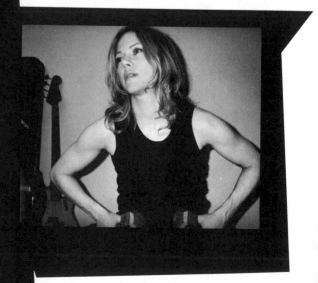

MAYBE YOU WANT TO LOSE weight or look good in a bathing suit. Maybe you want to be a professional wrestler or get a job busing tables or the kind of job that makes you pee into a cup. Maybe you just feel perpetually hungover and can't take it anymore. There are millions of reasons to make exercise a part of your life, and we've laid out a bunch more on page 152. We can spell them out for you, but at the end of the day, it's up to you to throw a mix on the stereo and work out. Knowing what you know now, why wouldn't you?

THINK ABOUT IT THIS WAY: fitness may give you the leading edge to pursue your vices with more vigor than Johnny Thunders, or it may inspire you to end them altogether. Whether you live on bacon burgers, smoke butts, drink like a fiend, say yes to drugs, or worship Satan, you'll have more fun doing all of it. Whether you plan to croak at thirty-five or a hundred and five, you simply cannot lose. We know that once you give it a try, you'll feel better—and that's the best motivation there is.

JOHNNY THUNDERS was originally born John Anthony Genzale, in 1952. Together with David Johansen, Jerry Nolan, Arthur Kane, and Sylvain Sylvain, they formed the cult band the New York Dolls in 1971. Playing rock 'n' roll influenced by MC5 and Iggy and the Stooges, they dressed in drag and were loud, snotty, and preceded the whole punk rock scene in NYC. They broke up after their second record, and Johnny started the band the Heartbreakers. Tragically, he died of a heroin overdose in 1991. He is one of the greatest punk rock guitar players that we can think of ... which is why we mention him so much in this book. Everyone wants to cover his song, "You Can't Put Your Arms Around a Memory." We love him, even though he probably would have kicked us in the face at one of his shows. We recommend checking out Born to Lose: The Last Rock and Roll Movie (1999), directed by Lech Kowalski, which includes interviews with Johnny's family, Dee Dee Ramone, and Stiv Bators. Johnny is forever remembered and lives on in everyone's rock 'n' roll life—whether they realize it or not.

Hate Mail

YOU CAN'T PLEASE EVERYONE. In fact, sometimes it's fun when you piss people off. A sampling of our detractors.

i hope iam not the first to tell you that you killed punk you trendy little mall rat girls who shop at hot topic

This makes me feel ashamed of being a punk. I really wanted to cry when I heard about this aweful mess of posers doing some skanking and moshing for exercise. Exercise? what? This is a disgrace to Punk and a disgrace to CBGB's. I have extreme hate for all of the people who participate in punk rock aerobics and even more for those who created it.

I printed you're website out and used it as toilet paper; maybe you could give me your address so I could send the poo to you.

SUBJECT: LISTEN UP YOU TRENDY F--KS
I HOPE YOUR F--KING COMPANY BLOWS THE F--K UP FOR KILLING THE TERM "PUNK." PUNK ISNT F--KING AEROBICS YOU DUMB FAT WHORE.

Just out of curiousity, do you really think that all other instructors that are not "punk instructors" are brain-dead bimbos in spandex thongs? I doubt you really do, but still, it's rather insulting ... Are you guys advocating health stuff or just fun? You said on your website "free your mind and your-butt-will follow." But your website and the article makes it look like a bunch of smoking boozers that just take a break to dance around a little. If that's the image you want ... okay! But it's not exactly a healthy one. How can a person addicted to tobacco or alcohol truly free his or her mind?

Who's idea was it to turn punk rock into a trendy workout? You f--ing poser punk rock bitches are all the same. What do you play at the classes? Blink-182? It's bad enough that punk rock is getting as trendy as it is. We dont need your help to get any bigger. Give it up ... for the sake of punk.

LOVE LETTERS

WHENEVER WE START TO WONDER if we've built a company from scratch for no good reason, we open the mailbox on our web site and drink in the adoration of our fans. Some of them have good punk stories of their own.

I think you and all the girls in P.R.A are really hot and some pictures of you all in the nude would be appreciated....yeah, it's a long shot, I know. But it's worth a try.

my name is federico (federick). i live in sud america (argentina), very punk land in the ass of the planet.
your idea of PRA is: wonderful. congratulation and good luck.
ps: i can not go to the aerobics—due to the ticket bus is too f--king expensive 4 me.
PS: dear maura you're a beatiful woman (i love your style baby, your attitude, and ... all) kiss-kiss for you (in your neck) god save the queeen!!!!

i am taking aerobics in my high school right now and, basically, it sucks ass!!!!! I asked my teacher if we could try out punk rock aerobics. She overwhelmingly said yes!!

I asked my P.E teacher could we POGO as an exercise in 1976!!

Hey I am totally interested in these classes and it sounds like a blast. However, I live in the total asshole of our country known as the midwest, and nothing remotely cool exists out here. Everything is based around having long blonde hair and wearing abercrombie out here...ugh.

Hi Hilken. I've never been to punk rock aerobics, but judging from your site, it rocks!... I teach hatha yoga at clubs around here (sometimes gentler stuff, and sometimes a bit more vigorous vinyasa type) and am looking for new venues. Have you ever thought about adding a yoga option to PRA?...I can see it now...guest musicians create an ethereal, meditative soundscape...candles, incense....Christmas lights.

hey! me and my friend r 14 and i saw PRA on MTV2 UltraSound ... we're dying to try it out cuz we love dancin @ shows and think it would be totally kick ass to do it as an exercise 2. ... so we were wondering if you have 2 b a certian age ... cuz if there isnt we'll deff be 2 a class durring r school vacation.

holy s--t, just lookin around the punk pages on the net and found THIS. so funny. punk s--t up
cheers
elvis von fan

TOP SIX PUNK ROCK PHYSIQUES

We tried to find ten. We were aghast to find there were only six worthy of inclusion.

1. HENRY ROLLINS Up next: The Men of Baywatch

2. GLENN DANZIG

3. IGGY POP So there, Surgeon General

4. KIM GORDON of Sonic Youth, roughly forty minutes after childbirth

5. IAN MACKAYE

6. JOAN JETT

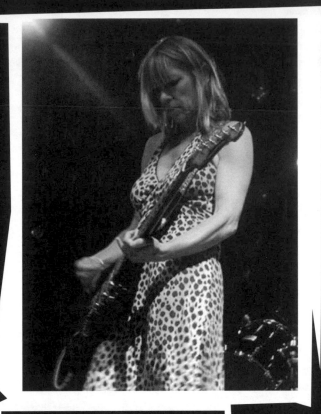

Kim Gordon

Henry Rollins

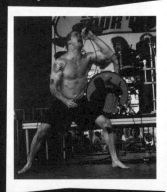

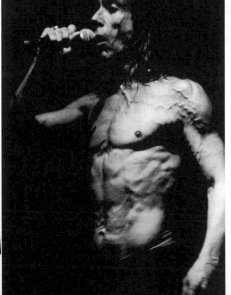

Iggy Pop

PUNK ROCK AEROBICS?

PRA IS THE HEIGHT of convenience for the laziest sods among you and will help take the edge off your boredom. You don't need a gym and can do this workout anywhere you want. Maybe you want to stay indoors with the shades drawn or be an exhibitionist and hang out with those Tai Chi weirdos at the park. You can bust out the jams in your bedroom, dorm room, squatters flat, or corporate office. You can do this workout alone, with friends, or even on a date (to break the ice, cut to the chase and start right in on the Slut Butt). Work out in your pajamas, birthday suit, best comfy stretch pants, or indulge in your secret fetish for leotards and sweatbands. You can do this workout at two in the afternoon or two in the morning when you stumble in from an evening of head-banging highjinks. You can listen to your favorite music at hearing-loss–inducing volumes, and when you're done (or even while you work out), you can enjoy a butt or a cold one.

BESIDES, IT'S FUNNY-LOOKING—and people who laugh supposedly live longer. We'll keep you from turning into a humorless old fart, with a big-ass chip on your fat, wattled shoulder. Even if you can't master the moves, you'll have a good time trying; for chrissakes, it's better than watching another episode of *Friends*. Even if the only exercise you get comes from flipping through the pages of this book, something in these pages is going to appeal to you, even if it's just a fine photograph of us demonstrating a Skank in all its clinical splendor.

Punk Rock Aerobics: stay alive to keep smashing things up!

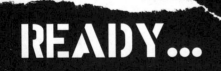

READY...

GETTING GEARED UP FOR YOUR WORKOUT

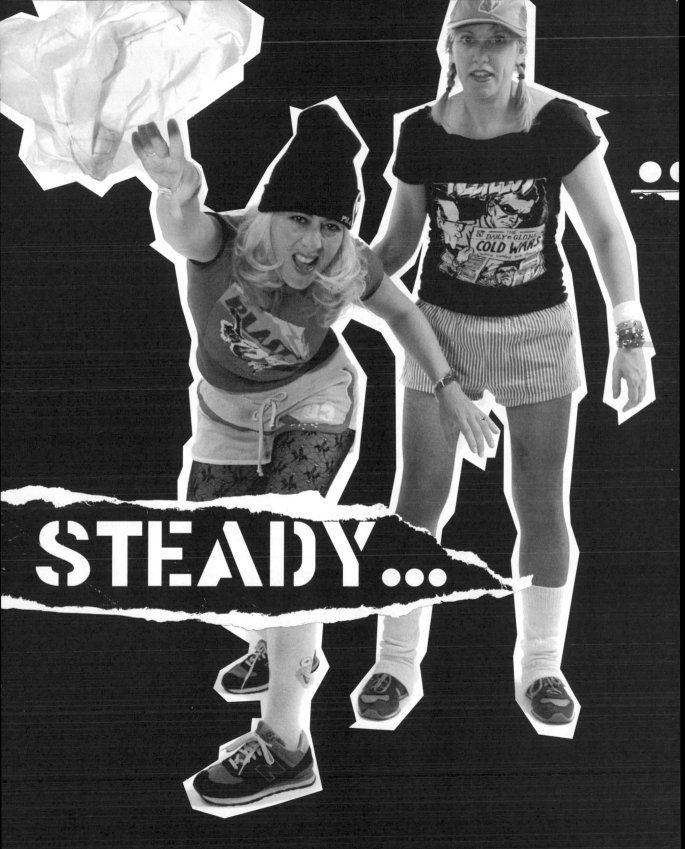

STEADY...

...GO!

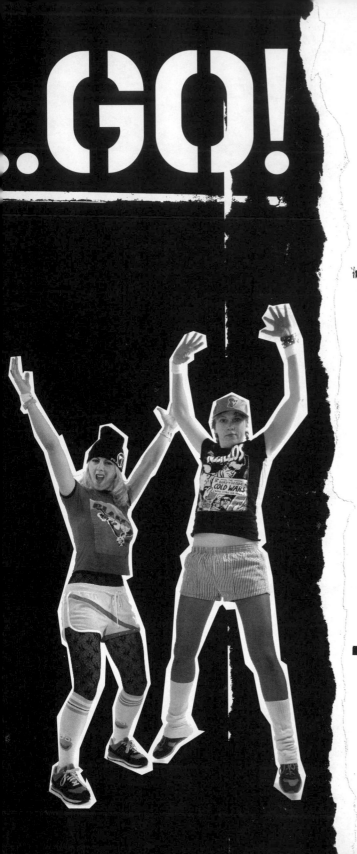

THE PRA WORKOUT does not necessitate a shopping spree at Foot Locker or Virgin Records. The equipment you need is limited and inexpensive, and it makes a big difference. We want to ensure that as soon as you start putting it all together PRA style, you'll be able to swan dive right into your workout. Don't freak out when we suggest what songs might work with what kind of moves, whether you're new to punk rock or just new to thinking about it as background music for strength training. Feel free to disagree with us about all matters musical. We know there's no such thing as an album list that doesn't start fights. You don't have to adhere to the letter of our law when it comes to anything else we say either, but you might find that your feet and shins start to complain if you ignore our advice on, say, sneakers.

REBELLIOUS JUKEBOX

THE SINGLE MOST IMPORTANT thing you need for your PRA workout is a stack of tunes: the more, the better. Some of you are no doubt sitting on a mountainous record collection worthy of the National Archives. Some of you are digging out your *Best of Blondie* CD and wondering how to pull this off. You don't need to be the rock geek who wrote papers on the Fall for the poetry unit in high school or even be a fan of punk. It's okay if you're just here to check it out. We'll give you some suggestions on how to get started.

We aren't snobs when it comes to music. We play all kinds of stuff in our class: Mission of Burma, the Slits, the Undertones, Killing Joke, Stiff Little Fingers, The Damned, Black Flag, The Only Ones, the Adverts, Eater, the Angry Samoans, Vice Squad, Siouxsie and the Banshees, Fugazi, Wire, Devo, Kraftwerk, and countless others. We also dig lots of newer music, like Sleater-Kinney, Erase Errata, the Thermals, Le Tigre, the White Stripes, and the Walkmen. We've put together a novel-length discography of all our favorite albums at the back of the book if you want to check it out online or at your nearest record store.

You will need to put together twenty-five to forty-five minutes of music on either a tape or CD. Or, if you're superlazy, just pick your favorite album and wing it. But we do think it's a lot more fun to have different songs.

IT'S LIKELY YOU'RE THINKING, "Geez, I haven't heard any of this stuff." So here's a list of indispensable punk rock compilations that will give you the information you need to hold your own at cocktail parties. Who knows, maybe they'll make you want to dig deeper; if they don't, who cares? Punk Rock 101 is not a prerequisite for PRA.

1. 1-2-3-4: PUNK AND NEW WAVE 1976–1979, IMPORT ONLY, 1999 (UNIVERSAL). 5-CD SET. The best punk rock CD box set available, this compilation is accompanied by a cool booklet providing a history lesson on each artist. It boasts a great variety of bands, from British punk and new wave to the New York scene. You can make all of your Punk Rock Aerobics workouts for the next ten years with just these five CDs. If you can get your hands on this one, go for it. You'll have a great time just putting it on the stereo and rocking out, and you'll get an education you couldn't otherwise get unless you were there at the time.

2. 60 CLASSIC PUNK TRACKS, VARIOUS ARTISTS, 2003, (SIMPLY THE BEST). 3-CD SET. This is a good initial investment in punk know-how in that there are probably more bands you've heard of than not. It only has three CDs, which is less of a commitment, and will inspire you with classic hard-to-find tunes such as "I'm Stranded" by The Saints and Generation X's "Ready Steady Go."

3. PUNK: THE WORST OF TOTAL ANARCHY, VARIOUS ARTISTS, 2001 (SIMPLY THE BEST). If you just want to check punk out to see if you like it rather than diving in headfirst, this is a fine choice—perfect for those who want to tread lightly in the land of punk.

YOU'LL BE PUTTING TOGETHER song lists for stretching, cardio, and weight and floor exercises. The following is what to look for.

STRETCHING

Five to ten minutes of music at the beginning and end of your cardio work. Stretching can be done to just about any music—we like Joy Division, Flipper, and some of the more droning bands that we can't indulge in when we are trying to get our heart rates up. But if you think you can do stretches to a handful of two-minute hardcore tunes, more power to you.

CARDIO

Twenty to forty minutes. Here's where you pick the tunes that transform you into a skanking, pogoing monster. Have fun and reach for all of your favorites. We suggest midtempo, pop-based stuff from the Clash, Buzzcocks, the Rezillos, or the Ramones. Don't worry, we'll turn a blind eye when you slip in the Go-Go's or Duran Duran.

STRENGTH TRAINING

Twenty minutes. Anything that helps you do your reps like an obedient robot is dandy. We love Iggy Pop! Hearing him is all the inspiration we need. Other bands that we've used for these exercises are Gang of Four, the Fall, Devo, and the Smiths. For those who think the Smiths and strength building don't mix, all we can do is swear by our experience. There's something to be said for the whiny voice of a pretty boy when you're doing biceps curls.

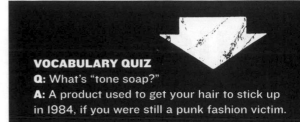

VOCABULARY QUIZ
Q: What's "tone soap?"
A: A product used to get your hair to stick up in 1984, if you were still a punk fashion victim.

* IT MIGHT BE HELPFUL TO USE 2 TAPES, ONE FOR YOUR STRETCHING AND STRENGTH TUNES, AND ONE FOR CARDIO TUNES. AFTER ALL, YOU DON'T WANT YOUR HEART RATE TO DROP WHILE YOU'VE GOT YOUR FINGER ON FAST FORWARD IN A MAD SEARCH FOR EXACTLY THE RIGHT IGGY POP SONG; IF YOU'RE BURNING A CD, ALL THE BETTER

RAGS, DUDS AND THREADS

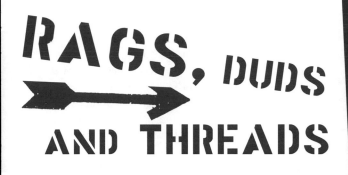

PEOPLE E-MAIL us all the time asking what to wear at our classes, and we always tell them, anything goes. The rule is that there are no rules. That's what makes it Punk Rock Aerobics. We've said before that it doesn't matter what you wear, and we don't care. But some things you probably shouldn't wear for practical reasons. You may be capable of figuring this out for yourself—jeans, for example. Bad idea. Or a stifling, J Lo–style terry cloth hookup. We like our hookups old school, Run DMC–style. They're a lot cooler and more comfortable. There are other things to consider: Should you wear that devastatingly ironic seventies iron-on tee with a plastic image stuck to the front that makes you sweat like Nixon on a lie detector, or a plain old cotton one? Should you risk wearing your favorite Ramones T-shirt and take the chance that sweat stains will forever ruin it (unless you regard stains as an enhancement), or wear one sporting the name of a forgotten indie band you liked for some reason in twelfth grade? It's your choice. We like to see people wear whatever makes them comfortable and lets them move around with ease; remember, this is not about fitting in. In our case, anyway, it's too late for that. Wear what makes you feel good. If we told you to show up with green hair and hot pink fishnets, we'd be huge dorks (and unnecessarily inconveniencing you). We've seen some pretty inspired getups (pajamas, for example, are surprisingly popular) and we never want to stifle anyone's creativity.

P.R.A. Q&A #4

Peaches
Sexy Electropunk Diva

Does Mike Watt's cycling regime make you want to go out and buy a bike?

Only if it's a bicycle built for two with Mike Watt.

Does Natalie Merchant's interpretive dancing inspire you?

Natalie Merchant gives interpretive dance a bad name.

Do you have a gym membership?

I'd like a membership to Jim Jarmusch.

If you exercise, what type of exercise do you do? And what kind of music do you listen to when working out?

I like to bike ride and sing Meatloaf's *Bat Out Of Hell*—the whole album really loud.

If you're on the road and one of your bandmates or fellow touring bands gets up to go for a jog, do you hate them or join them?

Just let 'em go. They'll be back.

Do you like your body, or are you among the ranks of people who think that if they could just lose those ten pounds, they'd be perfect?

i'm perfectly happy with my bloated stomach and my bye-bye wings and I especially like those cottage cheese patterns on my ass.

As a performer in the public eye, has body image ever been a concern? Have you ever had outside pressure (that is, from a label, etc.) about your weight/shape?

no i've made a career out of the opposite.

Do you think that fat people get no respect?

Fat people are hot. Haven't you heard that song "Kleine Dicker Junge" and "You're The One For Me Fatty"?

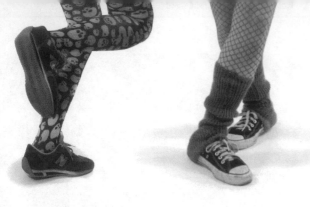

SNEAKERS

The only important thing you do need to wear in PRA are highly supportive sneakers. There really isn't any other shoe to wear when you're jumping up and down for twenty minutes at a stretch. Those Chucks are classic—and also your ticket to stress fractures and other impact-related injuries. Ditto for combat boots. We know Doc Martins are sometimes thought to possess the strange power to blend with any social situation, but this is one occasion for which they are not suitable.

And you don't need to work an extra shift to buy sneakers: Saucony makes a decent shoe for about $30. If you find a pair of vintage Reeboks, you'll be cooler than a Klondike Bar. Cooler yet, you could sell the Reeboks on eBay to some *Vogue* editor, then take the money and buy yourself a really nice pair of sneakers! That would be punk. We love the old-school New Balance. I guess we love the old school in general.

WEIGHTS

Talk about being cheap; as mentioned earlier, start-up money for this enterprise came from unemployment checks, which means no extravagance. So we bought bricks at Home Depot and spray-painted them. They work great. It's a little tricky to get a grip on 'em, but perfect for our budget and perfect for beginners, because they only weigh between three and five pounds. We suggest using whatever weight feels right for you. If you're a beginner at this whole workout thing, we suggest going to your local sporting goods store and buying three-pound weights for starters. Bricks will do the trick if you're not sure whether you'll ever want to work out again and want to see how it goes before you make an investment. A couple of full two-liter soda bottles work fine; just keep the caps screwed on tight, obviously. Remember, there's always an object around your house that you can use—pick up the keg that you never returned to the liquor store, the baby, or the TV. As you find your inner Lou Ferrigno (the original Hulk), you will upgrade.

A few months after holding these classes, we happened to be flipping through *Mojo* magazine. They did an interview with Chuck Berry in which he was quoted as saying that one of the things he did for exercise was to lift bricks in his garage. It was like the granddaddy of rock 'n' roll putting his stamp of approval on PRA. We cut out a photo of him and taped it on our wall, along with one of our favorite advertising slogans, "Face it: Your gym sucks." It was a great moment for PRA, a moment of communion with our brick-lifting ancestors. Go, Chuck, go.

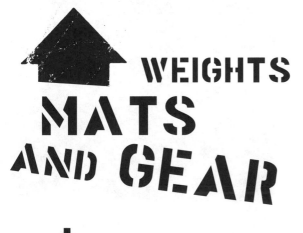

WEIGHTS MATS AND GEAR

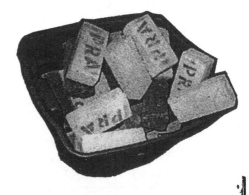

MAT

Okay, maybe some of you think that it would be way more punk for us not to use a mat—especially since rock clubs are famous for stamped-out cigarettes and wads of spit right next to your head. But most of us prefer a little more support and would rather work out under less stomach-turning conditions. Eventually, you will definitely need some kind of padded surface for the floor exercises.

For the class, we started buying slabs of rubber foam—they're cheap and had the perfect look. But after a class or two, they were a little too dirty to use anymore and it didn't seem like proper hygiene, although most of our students didn't seem to mind. So we went to a few wholesale places to buy rolls of foam and cut them into long rectangular pieces as people came to our classes. They come in cool colors like pink and red, but we soon realized that they were getting as filthy as the foam we used earlier, only you couldn't see the dirt as well. So now we have real mats for class. Yes, one could even call them yoga mats—wanna say something about it?

So cave in and buy a mat, unless in the comfort of your own home you can lay down a rug or towel. If you can't afford a mat, we suggest beach towels, carpeting, carpet liner, or foam— whatever provides the most comfort for you while you work out on the floor. Sure, some of you are too punk for that; do exercises on a hard wood floor—a pool table, for all we care.

WATER

Make sure there's plenty of it. Especially if you're planning on doing our two twenty-minute rock blocks, broken up with strength training. You have to be hydrated to keep from passing out. In our classes, we always provide water for people; it's important. We strongly suggest drinking it between each cardio and strength-training section. You should never do a PRA workout without some sips. (On one occasion in England, the sips were straight from a 40 ounce, but you should probably do that kind of sipping after your workout; we needed extra inspiration that day.)

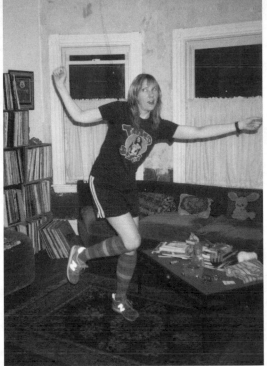

Maura rocking out at home

FLOOR

About that floor you're about to pogo on: we hope you guys all know that concrete does not an exercise floor make. We like natural surfaces; find one that's made out of wood. In a pinch, linoleum will do. Your shag-carpeted living-room is a decent last resort. It's all about the knees and shin splints. Ignore us at your peril.

SPACE

Give yourself a little. You need room to maneuver. When we first started this, we were cramped in our living room and when we found real space to work in, it made a huge difference. The more floor space you get, the longer the moves, the leaner the muscles—the bigger, the better. Push that coffee table or couch out of the way and rock the roof off.

2

DON'T BE A

STRETCHING

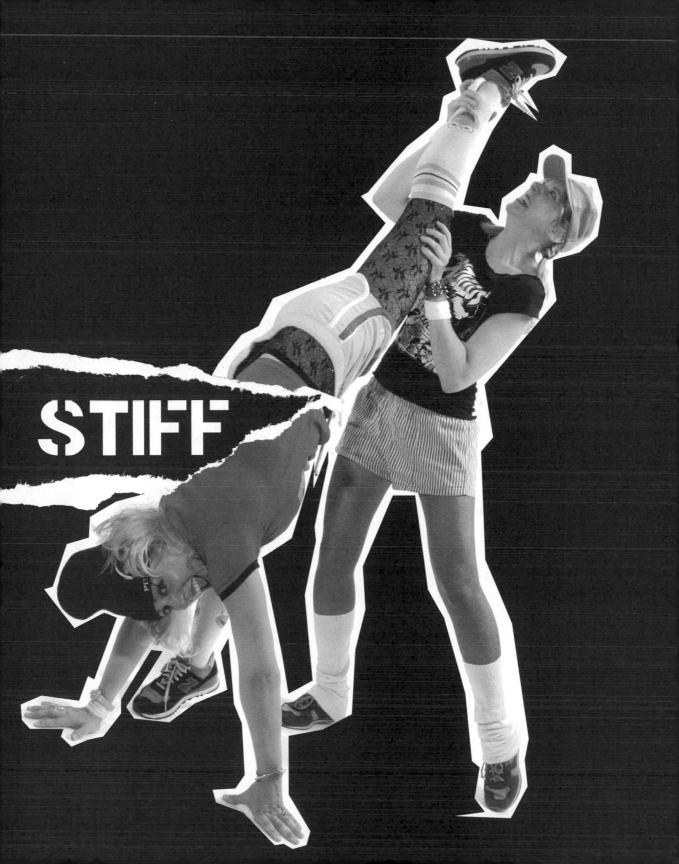

STIFF

HERE ARE SOME TIPS TO KEEP IN MIND WITH ANY STRETCH:

- Hold each stretch for ten seconds and add more time as you become more flexible

- Don't start bouncing into the stretch—it may be tempting when you're listening to the Clash's "White Riot" for the first time in twenty years, but you could overextend yourself and pull a muscle

- If something feels painful or entirely wrong, it probably is—stop and adjust your form until your body sends you the message that you're doing it right.

EVEN IF YOU KNOW MORE ABOUT EXERCISE than we did when we started—which is to say, anything—it's probably safe to assume you don't know jack about stretching. By the time you finally do try to haul your ass off the couch, chances are good that you feel as though rigor mortis has set in. But before you begin this or any other workout, it's important to stretch. It's even more important to get stretching after you're done with your workout and your muscles are warmed up.

If you think that stretching is stupid and want to blow it off, you better be ready to familiarize yourself with all the creams at the local pharmacy for sports injuries, and maybe retain a manservant to buckle your belt and tie your shoelaces. Although there is disagreement in the fitness world over whether or not stretching truly prevents injury, we can tell you this: whenever we blew it off, we were crying into a vat of Tiger Balm the next day. Stretching has been proven to improve flexibility, posture, and relieve tension. It helps to keep your muscles in balance so that you don't strain or overuse the wrong ones when you summon enough discipline to work out. What does this mean for you? It means that the next time you bend down to pick up that case of beer, you won't wince like an old man.

Flexibility is something you can improve and develop, but it's also something you're born with. You know the old trick where you roll up your tongue like a burrito? Some people can do it and some can't—you either have it or you don't. We won't bore you with details, but it has to do with elastic properties in your ligaments. You can work on stretching them out, but some people simply have more of them. Other factors that affect flexibility are age and whether or not you spend your entire waking life sitting in front of a screen.

In our classes, we like to do eight to twelve minutes of stretching so that we can be fully prepared to rock ourselves into a frenzy. To get started, we will show you some basic warm-up stretches. Some of our cardio moves can put you through the wringer, so you don't want to dive in headfirst with a stiff neck. When you're done working out, stretching can help you cool off so that you're not raging through the streets red faced and panting like a maniac. You also get more out of your stretches at the end because your body is warmed up and more limber; and remember, you can do these stretches anytime. Whether you're bored doing dishes at the kitchen sink or too busted to do an actual workout, it always helps to stretch. It's possible to do too many jumps or too many crunches, but it's impossible to spend too much time stretching.

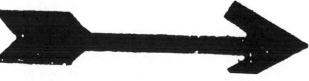

WARM-UP
LOWER BODY STRETCHES

One thing you gotta love about yoga: the evocative names they give those poses. In homage to our hippie colleagues, we named all of our stretches too. You may recognize some of these by another name, but we like to think of them by their glam rock names.

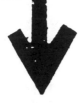

MONO LEG

quadriceps (front of thigh)

WE HEARD THROUGH the grapevine that if you lift up your free arm while doing this stretch, you will achieve something similar to what's known in yoga as **Tree Pose**. This is the lazy no-arm version.

- Stand, facing straight ahead with both feet placed on the floor.

- Bend up your back leg, grab your foot and hold it, pressing it against your butt.

- Hold for ten seconds.

- Release and repeat with the other leg.

Do this twice on each side.

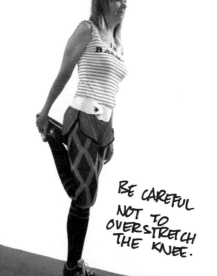

BE CAREFUL NOT TO OVERSTRETCH THE KNEE.

* KEEP GOOD POSTURE WHILE DOING THIS EXERCISE. KEEP ABS TIGHTLY HELD IN.

UNNATURAL AXE

hamstring (back of thigh)

- Stand facing straight.

- Bring your left leg straight out and rest it on its heel.

- Flex the toes of your left foot up toward the ceiling.

- Bend your right leg and sit back, putting weight onto the right foot, and hinge the torso forward.

- Keep bending and lean the torso slightly forward until you feel a stretch at the back of your left leg.

- Hold the position for ten seconds.

- Release and repeat on other leg.

Do this twice on each side.

* REMEMBER TO SQUARE THE HIPS AND SHOULDERS WITH THE LEG YOU ARE STRETCHING.

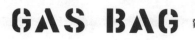
GAS BAG

gastrocnemius/soleus (calves)

DON'T BE SURPRISED if this movement has you passing wind.

- Stand in a staggered lunge position with your left knee bent, right leg straight behind you, heel on floor.

- Arms on hips or on your leg, above your knee.

- Bend your front leg so that your knee is directly above your ankle.

- Press gently forward with your hips and bend the front knee deeper.

- Feel the stretch in your back leg calf.

- Hold the position for ten seconds.

  Do this twice with each leg.

MORON ROLLUP

tibialis anterior (ankles and shins)

ROLL IT UP, roll it down, ROLL IT UP, roll it down.

- Stand in a staggered lunge position with your front knee bent, back leg straight behind you, heel on floor.

- Your back foot is flat on the ground, hands on hips.

- Slowly roll your back foot up and down, only rolling up to the ball of your foot.

Repeat this ten times on each side.

LOOSE
UPPER BODY STRETCHES

BACK SCRATCHER

triceps (back of the arm)

CLOSE YOUR EYES and imagine a huge rash spreading across your back, and you can't itch it—get that hand back there, you can do it.

- Stand facing straight ahead. Drop your chin down to your chest. Reach your right arm straight up overhead, palm forward.

- Bend your elbow and drop your right hand to the back of your neck, palm facing in.

- Reach overhead with your left arm and grasp just below your right elbow. With your left hand, gently pull the right arm to the left. Feel the stretch in the back of the right upper arm.

- Hold the position for ten seconds.

Release and repeat on other arm two times each.

CAT SCRATCH FEVER

trapezius/latissimus dorsi/erector spinae (back)

THIS ONE will make you feel as though you are auditioning for a third-rate version of Cats ... Meoww.

- Stand facing straight ahead.

- Lower your torso so that your back is flat and horizontal and your hands are resting above your knees.

- Keeping your back straight, make sure your knees are slightly bent, directly under your hips.

- Slowly curl your back into a hump.

- Slowly flatten your back and return to the starting position.

  Repeat this move five times.

- Slowly roll back up into your starting position.

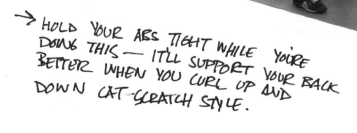

→ HOLD YOUR ABS TIGHT WHILE YOU'RE DOING THIS — IT'LL SUPPORT YOUR BACK BETTER WHEN YOU CURL UP AND DOWN CAT-SCRATCH STYLE.

DELTOID VOID

deltoids (shoulders)

FEEL LIKE your arms have an uncontrollable urge.

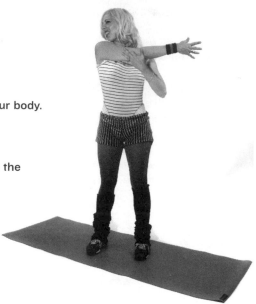

- Stand facing straight ahead.

- Bring arm up sideways and toward the midline of your body.

- Swing arm horizontally forward and grab it.

- Hold it to your chest, pulling gently. Turn and look in the opposite direction of your arm.

- Hold the position for ten seconds.

- Release and repeat on other arm.

   Do this twice on each side.

LEANING TOWER OF TORSO

external obliques/deltoid (side of stomach and back)

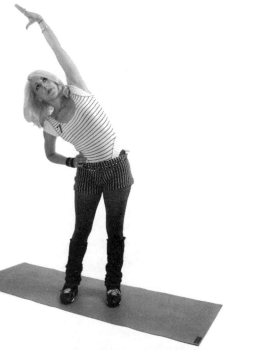

DON'T WORRY, you won't fall over—unless your equilibrium is out of whack from a night of head-banging hi-jinks.

- Stand facing straight, with your feet shoulder-width apart.

- Place your right hand on your hip for support and reach your left arm up and overhead.

- Gently bend your torso over.

- Feel the stretch up through your left side.

- Hold the position for ten seconds.

   Do this twice on each side.

18 | P.R.A.

NECK BREAKA

trapezius (neck)

AS YOU ROLL YOUR HEAD, listen for that crackling sound—that is the sound of old age.

- Stand facing straight ahead, with your feet shoulder-width apart.

- Drop your chin down to your chest.

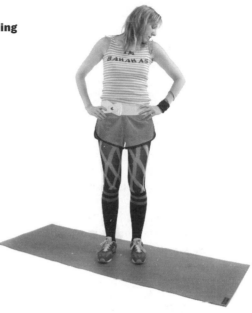

- Keeping your chin down close to your body, roll your neck from shoulder to shoulder in a smooth controlled motion, 180 degrees.

- Roll your neck from side to side ten times.

Rest and repeat.

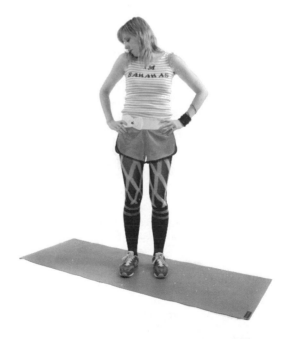

ROCK 'N' ROLLER

trapezius/rhomboids/latissimus dorsi/hamstring group
(upper back, middle back, rib cage, back of legs)

- Stand facing straight ahead with your feet shoulder-width apart.

- Starting with the top of your head, slowly roll down, knees slightly bent as you go. Roll all the way down as far as you can, one vertebrae at a time. Try to touch your fingertips to the floor.

- Now that you're hanging down there and getting a head rush, shake everything out.

- You should feel your whole torso, head, shoulders, and hands all at once shake out, bringing relief of tension and tightness. Now stop the rock and slowly roll back up...one vertebrae at a time.

wOW...

...these LeGwArMers lOOk reAlLy gOOd wItH THEse tiGhTs.

RIPPED T-SHIRT STRETCH

trapeziums/rhomboids/latissimus dorsi/medial and posterior deltoid/rotator cuff
(upper and lower back)

YOU KNEW there was a reason you never threw away that shredded, worn-out Necros T-shirt ...

- Stand facing straight ahead.

- With the ripped T-shirt in your left hand, lift it up over your head and bend it back behind your head.

- Bend the right arm behind your back and bring it up so that it can reach and grasp the other end of the T-shirt. Hold it there for ten seconds.

- Slowly move your hands closer together by crawling them up or down the T-shirt. Hold it there again for ten seconds.

Switch sides and repeat with the other arm.

THE GOAL IS TO INCH YOUR HANDS CLOSER EACH TIME UNTIL THEY EVENTUALLY TOUCH.

REAL TIME COOL
BODY STRETCHES
TO COOL DOWN

A lot of these are done on the floor, so whip out your mat or maybe a smelly old down parka from your closet, and lay your body down.

AB FLAB

LOOK, mA. no doUBLe ChiN!

THERE'S A GREAT episode of Ab Fab in which Patsy and Edina get all punked out to go to a Marilyn Manson concert. Patsy looks particularly special—right up there with the photos of Liz Hurley as a teenage punk.

- Lie face down on the mat.

- Your palms are face down on the mat, under your shoulders. Pull yourself up, placing your weight directly onto your elbows.

- Arch the back slightly and keep your head in line with the spine. Feel the stretch through the abdominal muscles.

- Hold the position for ten seconds.

Rest and repeat. Do this twice.

HAM SANDWICH STRETCH

hamstrings (back of thigh)

- Lie on your back, knees bent and feet flat on the floor, hip-width apart. Straighten and lift your right leg (knee slightly bent). Hold both hands around the right leg.

- Keep shoulders and hips on the mat as you gently pull the right leg toward you. Feel the stretch in the back of your upper right leg.

- Hold the position for ten seconds.

- Release and repeat with the other leg.

Do this twice on each side.

PArDon mE, do yOu hAVE Any GREY POupON?

SPINAL TWIST

erector spinae lattimus dorsi/medius (upper and lower back, hip)

TWIST IT to II ... rock on.

- Sit straight up with the left leg straight. Cross your right leg over the left leg.

- Using your left elbow, gently push against the outside of your right knee. Slowly rotate your upper body to the right, pushing with the left arm.

- Hold the position for ten seconds.

- Release and repeat with the other leg.

Do this twice on each side.

gEe, my AsS FEeLS tErRIFIc!

* DO THIS EXERCISE SLOWLY AND CAREFULLY.

LEGS McNEIL

erector spinae, lattimus dorsi, gluteus meduis, trapezius
(upper and lower back, hips, ass, neck)

- Lie flat on your back. Bend and bring the right leg up and hold it to your chest with both hands.

- Turn the bent leg to the left, aiming the knee to the floor. At the same time, bring your right arm out to the right side to support you.

- Allow your upper body to naturally twist around as your left hand presses your right knee into the ground. Turn your head to the right arm that is out and supporting you.

- Hold the position for ten seconds. Release and repeat on the other side.

Do this twice on each side.

LA RESTE

erector spinae (lower back)

This is one of those relaxing moves to bring your blood pressure down to the nearly dead.

- Lie down on your back.

- Bend the knees and slowly bring your legs up to your chest.

- Put your arms around your bent legs and pull them closer to the chest.

- Press your lower back into the mat; feel the stretch.

- Hold the position for ten seconds.

Repeat.

※ DO WHATEVER WORKS BEST TO MAKE YOU FEEL YOUR LOWER BACK RELEASE TENSION AND PRESS INTO THE MAT.

→ SOMETIMES IT HELPS TO CROSS YOUR FEET AT THE ANKLES.

BOOTLICKER

deltoids, lattimus dorsi (shoulders, lower back)

GET DOWN and lick my shiny Docs, you pussy.

• Kneel down on the mat.

• Sit back, moving your butt toward the heels of your feet.

• Extend your arms out in front of your body, elbows straight, palms pressing down into the mat.

• Feel the stretch through the upper arms, shoulders, lower back, and abdominal muscles.

• Hold the position for ten seconds.

Release and repeat.

* SUPPORT YOURSELF WITH YOUR HANDS AS YOU SLOWLY SLIDE DOWN AND ASSUME THE POSITION, ESPECIALLY THOSE OF YOU WITH BAD BACKS

AT LOOSE ENDS

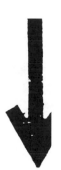

Despite our best efforts to provide you with the most perverse workout philosophy in America, we sometimes find ourselves outdone by the real fitness professionals. Here are a few stretches we've gleaned from apparently serious workout literature:

I SEE SPIDERS

THIS IS ONE move that comes naturally to those of you who surpass butts and booze in your ah, chemical intake. If you go to New York City, you'll notice its popularity among many individuals lying on the floor of Penn Station.

- Open your hand as if you're about to smack somebody.

- Briskly smack yourself upside the head.

- Repeat the same maneuver on other parts of your body, such as your legs, arms, and chest.

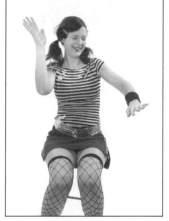
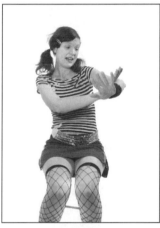

Indie rock princess Mary Timony came by for this one.

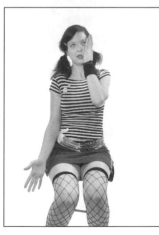
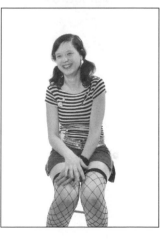

THIS WORKS BE-
CAUSE SOMETIMES
YOU HAVE TO
SLAP YOURSELF OUT
OF IT. YOU'LL SEE,
TRY IT.

PUT A CORK IN IT

THIS ONE is a great stretch to loosen your jaw. Unless you know someone who can give you the Heimlich maneuver, we recommend that you use a thermos cap instead of a cork (**T.D.** insisted on wine)—and definitely don't try this alone.

- Remove the cap from a thermos—a wine cork is too small in circumference. Hold it in your mouth between your teeth.

- Keep it there until your jaw experiences relief.

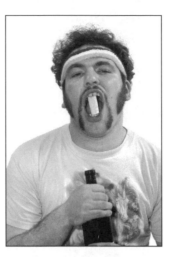
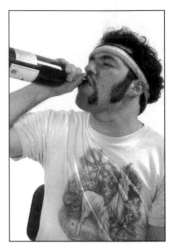

THE GENE SIMMONS

ELSEWHERE this has been called Yoga Lion Pose. We can't imagine what it has to do with yoga, or with any great cat other than Peter Kriss.

- Stand with your back straight.

- Open your mouth wide.

- Stick your tongue out as far as possible.

- Open your eyes wide.

- Breathe in, then breathe out, making a noise like haaah.

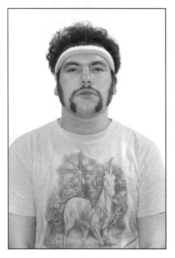
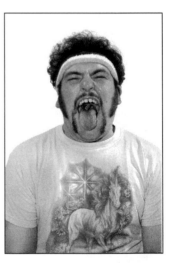

P.R.A. Q&A #5

Peter Prescott

Drummer for Mission of Burma

....

Does Mike Watt's cycling regimen make you want to go out and buy a bike?

I don't know, but I've had a bike for at least the last fifteen years. It's one of the few forms of exercise I get. It's not for the exercise, though. It's motivated by hatred of the bus and train.

Were you ever the last one to get picked for kickball in grade school? Did you ever get a doctor's note so you wouldn't have to take gym class?

I played kickball. I wasn't a total couch potato.

What songs or records have inspired you to physically move?

"I Get Wet" by Andrew WK. It's the industrial pogo music. It would be perfect for your class.

When you go on the road, do you lose weight or gain weight?

Gain weight. You're in the van, reading or getting stoned.

Is skinny better than buff?

To me, yes. And I don't mean excessively. It's the rock mentality, the old rock mentality. That indie rock, hopelessly skinny body. I think excessive body attention is narcissistic. I think it means you're spending too much time looking in the mirror.

Do you think that fat people get no respect?

(Disrespect) happens, whether you have a funny nose, or you're losing hair, like some of us. Whether you want to or not you judge people before they've spoken. That sucks that people operate that way. I try not to think that way.

Are you afraid of dodgeball?

No. It was a fun school activity.

P.R.A. Q&A #6

John Doe

Singer and Guitarist for X,
The Mighty Punk Rock Band

....

Were you ever the last one to get picked for kickball in grade school? Did you ever get a doctor's note so you wouldn't have to take gym class?

I swam, soccer, wrestling and lacrosse until rock, girls and drugs (11th grade).

Do you think William S. Burroughs ever lifted a weight in his life?

Obviously heroin either kills you or keeps you young.

Does Richard Simmons make you laugh or make you think of a scary clown?

Cute. Good for pissing off homo-phobes.

Has your state of "being in shape" ever effected your performance either positively or negatively? Do you tend to work up a sweat on stage?

Sweat? Bonebrake and I have "wringing out T-shirt" contests. Recently quit drinking before X shows and jog thirty to forty-five minutes while on tour.

3

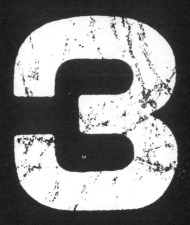

KiCK OUT

CARDIO MOVES

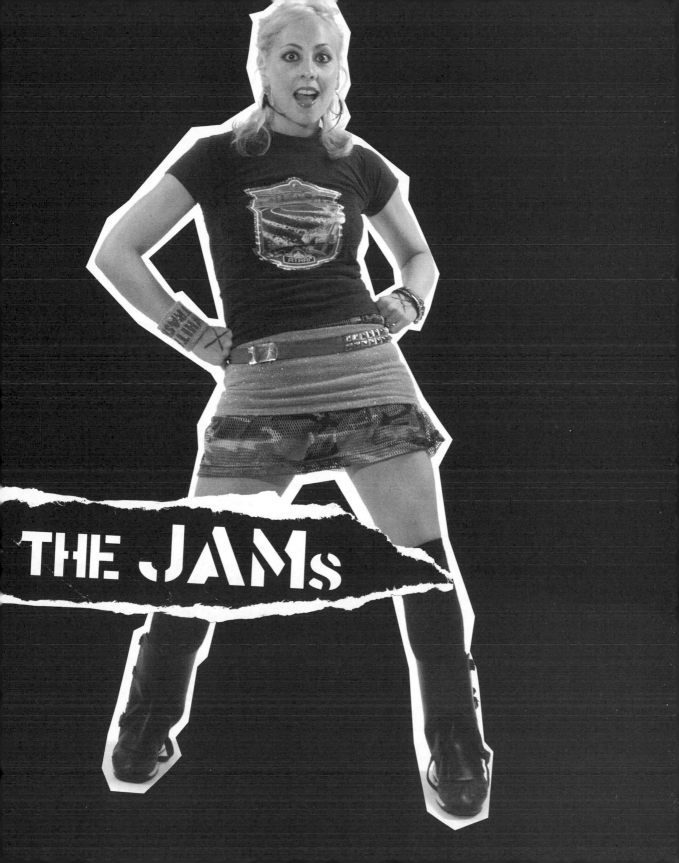

THE JAMs

ONCE YOU START ROCKING the cardio, never again will you believe a rock star who tells an interviewer that he sits in an armchair all day sipping Night Train Express. Running around onstage is a strenuous workout. Factor in the singing and screaming and partying the night before and it becomes clear that they really do deserve the big bucks and adoration of millions—they are also either young or in fantastic shape.

Cardio's not easy. This is the stuff that leaves you panting, sweating, and feeling as though you might collapse. Obviously, it's a lot easier to chill on the couch watching reruns of KOJAK. But with cardio, you'll build a stronger heart that pumps greater volumes of oxygenated blood without having to work as hard. This means that you'll reduce the chances of having a heart attack in the middle of a pogo session in your living room.

THE MOVES: HI-FI AND LO-FI

There are tons of easy and fun moves in the PRA workout to help warm your cold, cold hearts. Most of the time we don't care if you do them correctly. As long as you're moving, you're doing yourself a favor. When in doubt, you can always pogo. Besides, this isn't about scoring a perfect 10 at the next *Flashdance* contest.

The moves in the PRA workout are divided into Hi-Fi and Lo-Fi levels of exertion, and on a one to three scale of diehard difficulty (indicated by skull and crossbones). We will define the moves, and later, we will show you how to combine them to build a complete and personalized cardio workout, something we like to call *combo-hatching*.

Lo-Fi is the PRA dummy term for low-impact aerobics—that is, aerobic exercises done with one foot on the floor at all times. This means less impact, less pounding on your body. It's not necessarily a lower-intensity workout; your heart rate will remain elevated enough to make a difference. It's easier on the joints, resulting in fewer aches and pains. Eliminating forms of repetitive jumping—such as constant jogging—reduces the risk of stress on joints, tendon overuse, injury, and shin splints.

Hi-Fi is (duh) the PRA dummy term for high-impact aerobics—that is, aerobic exercises during which *both* feet leave the floor at the same time (activities such as jogging, hopping, or pogoing). High-impact aerobics are more intense, and your heart rate will definitely be raised to its highest working level. Hi-Fi feels a lot like getting jacked up at a show and pogoing your brains out.

It doesn't matter which you choose, because both Hi-Fi and Lo-Fi moves are extremely effective at bringing your heart rate up so that your body is working hard enough for you to break a sweat.

BASIC, FOOTLOOSE, AND PRIME MOVERS

We've further divided these into three types: Basic, Footloose, and Prime Movers. Once you understand the similarities between moves that are in the same group, they're easier to learn. They're listed from easy to hard—and when you see the skull and crossbones, you better beware!

BASIC

These are the moves that you simply can't live without. They're easy, and you can do them to almost any song. You can even pick one and do it through an entire song—but since most of them are Hi-Fi moves, they might leave you missing your old pal, oxygen.

POGO

THIS IS THE PRA EQUIVALENT OF CLASSIC COKE. It's the most accessible, coolest, most versatile and fun move ever. It's Punk Rock Aerobics for Dummies! Do we really need to explain this one to you?

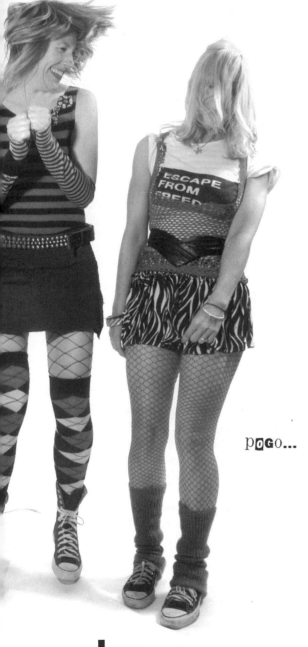

pOGo...

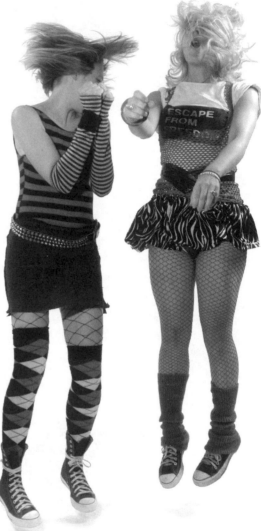

1 Jump up and down like you are on a pogo stick.

Move the rest of your body however you want. Go nuts while you jump in rhythm to the music.

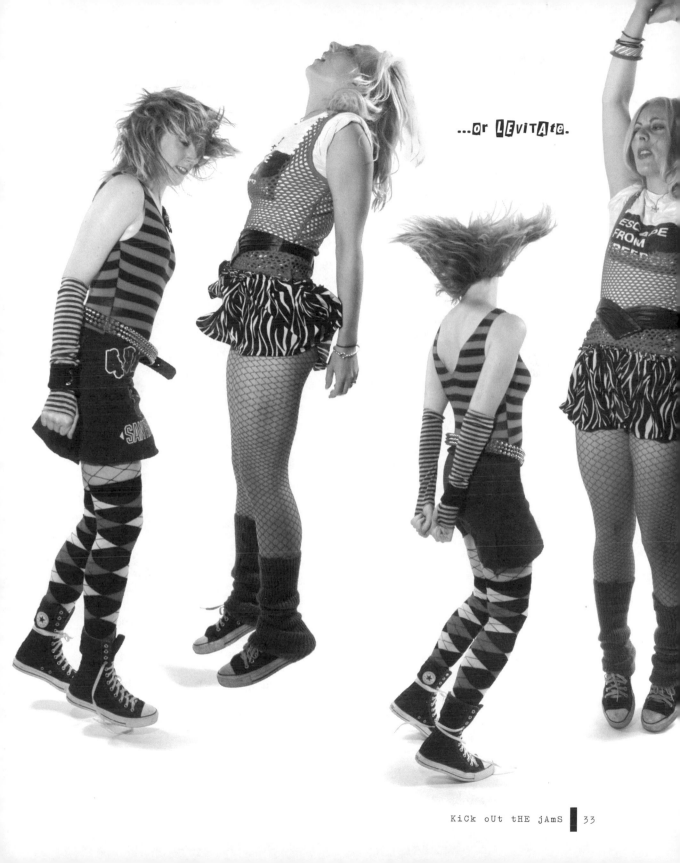

...or LEVITATE.

SKANK

FOR THIS ONE, our Punk Rock Aerobics instructor Ama channeled those skinheads from the pit. Make it as aggressive as you can—if you're familiar with the drawing of the punk kid on Circle Jerks records, imitate him and you'll be all set.

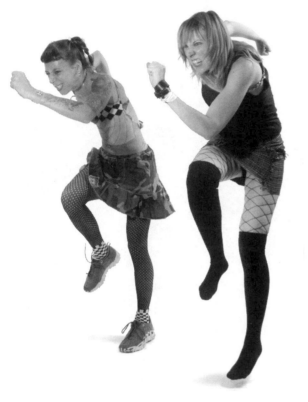

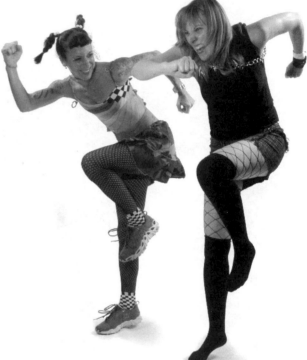

1 Make fists with your hands.

Move your arms and legs as if marching in place.

2 Make the movements big and aggressive, bringing your arms and knees up much higher.

Jump with each swing of the arms and legs.

Rock your head back and forth.

ROCK

 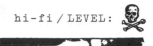

WE LOVE to scream ROCK! and launch right into this move. Maybe that's because you don't have to be Baryshnikov to pull it off.

I'M A JOKER, I'M A SMOKER, I'M A MIDNIGHT TOKER...

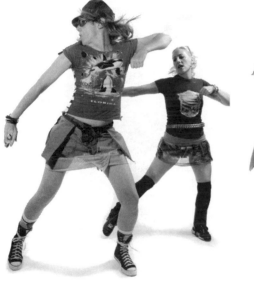
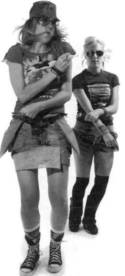
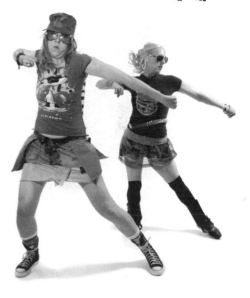

1 Face forward and jump your legs apart like you're doing a jumping jack, but throw your weight to one side of your body.

2 Jump back to starting position.

3 Now do the same thing, throwing your weight to the other side.

Throw in the arms as you go from side to side, bringing them in and out in whatever fashion rocks your world the hardest.

WACK JACK

 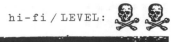

A JUMPING JACK, only whacked—don't think about it, just shut up and do as we say.

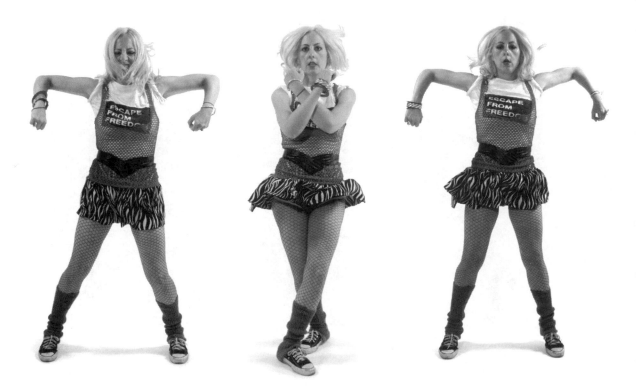

1 Stand facing straight ahead, and jump both feet to the side (as you would for a regular jumping jack).

As both legs go out to the side, lift your arms up and out at your sides, with your hands facing down

2 Jump and cross your feet with arms in, one in front of the other.

3 Jump back out and in again (crossing the arms and feet the other way, if you like).

→ REMEMBER, WHEN YOU JUMP OUT TO THE SIDE, YOUR KNEES SHOULD NEVER COMPLETELY STRAIGTEN. YOU COULD HURT YOUR KNEES THAT WAY...

...AND THE LAST THING YOU WANT IS TO EXPLAIN TO YOUR DATE THAT YOU HURT YOURSELF WACK JACKIN'.

CROSS-CROSS

 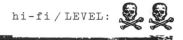

THIS MOVE WAS inspired by the Teen Idles' EP "Minor Disturbance (Too Young to Rock)." The record cover shows two fists crossed at the wrist, with giant Xs scrawled on them. It's easy, it's fun, and you don't need to be "straight edge" to master it. Think of this as cheerleading for punks.

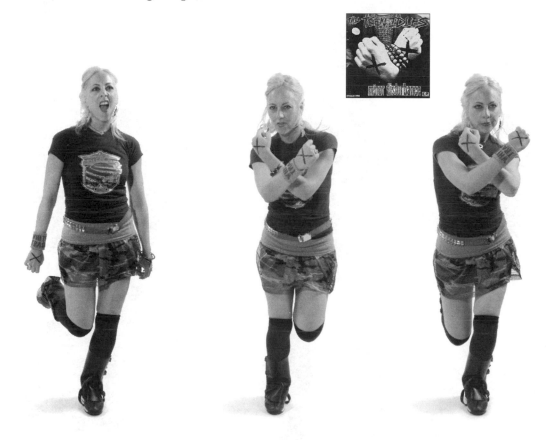

1 Jog in place.

2 Make fists with your hands and cross your arms in front of your chest, forming an X.

3 Cross the arms right over left and left over right, quickly, for two counts, then lower for two counts.

* AS YOU JOG, IT HELPS TO THINK IN 4/4 TIME (SO PUNK ROCK!): CROSS, CROSS, ONE, TWO.

GO-GO

NO, WE ARE NOT trying to make you look like some Coyote Ugly girl dancing on a bar somewhere. Dig out Agent Orange's cover of the Ventures' classic "Pipeline" for this one.

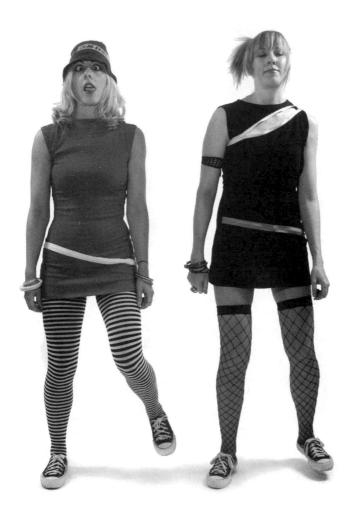

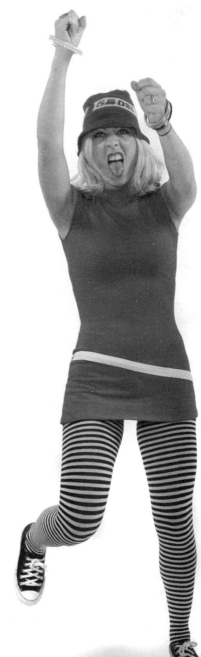

1 Start with your feet shoulder-width apart.

Shift your weight from side to side like a go-go dancer, bending your knees as you go.

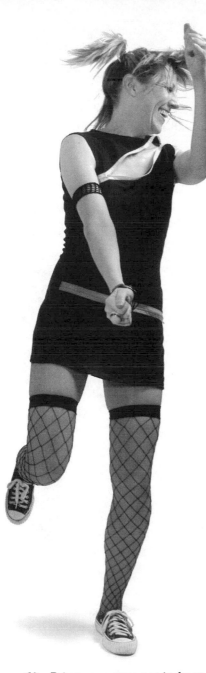

GOOD thINg We BOuGHt THAt go-go AeROBICs vIdeO!

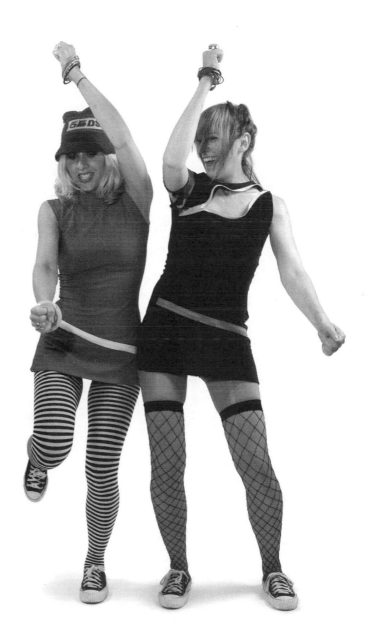

2 Bring your arms out in front of you and start swinging them up and down to the beat.

Throw in a subtle twist of the hips and shoulders, and you're good to go-go.

SIDESWIPE

ONCE YOU HAVE IT DOWN, the Sideswipe can be fun, and is also an awesome cooldown move. Feel free to add arm movements, punching the air or reaching up over your head. Make this one your own—give it all the oomph you can muster, and do it as fast or slow as you want.

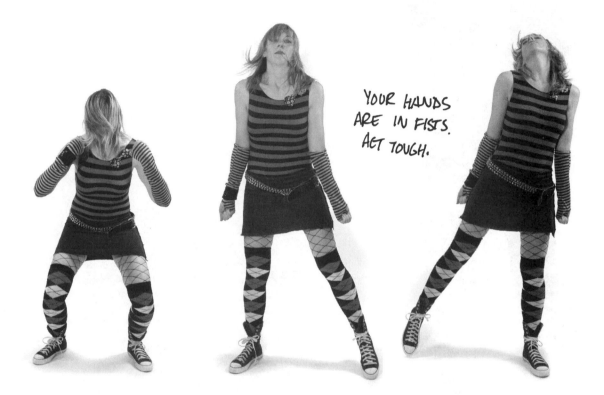

YOUR HANDS ARE IN FISTS. ACT TOUGH.

1 Stand facing straight ahead with both feet placed a little wider than shoulder-width apart, hands at your sides.

Bend your knees and elbows, bringing your hands up to the shoulders.

2 Now straighten your arms and legs, and as you do, lean to one side, putting all your weight on one foot.

Return to your starting position, knees bent, hands raised to the shoulders.

3 Push off to the other side.

Rock side to side, always bringing your arms up and down with each movement.

BACNE

 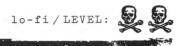

THIS ONE HAS US SCREAMING, "back, knee, back, knee, back, knee!" when we do it in class ... we sound as if we are chanting to the god of hairy pimples.

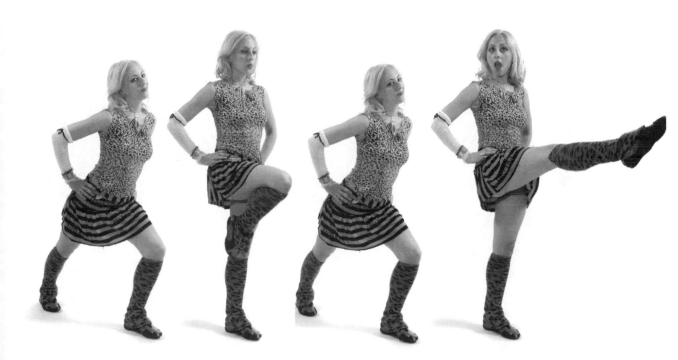

1 Stand facing straight ahead, hands on hips, right leg back so that you are in a lunging position.

Your weight should be evenly distributed on both feet.

2 Raise your right knee as high as you can.

3 Bring it back to its starting position.

4 Now kick the right leg out in front of you (waist level, at the most).

Repeat the same pattern five times. Switch to the other leg and repeat.

✻ YOUR ARMS CAN BE WHEREVER YOU WANT.
YOU CAN NOW OFFICIALLY SAY, "I HAVE BACNE."

CIRCLE JOG

MAKE USE of those Circle Jerk records if you've got 'em...

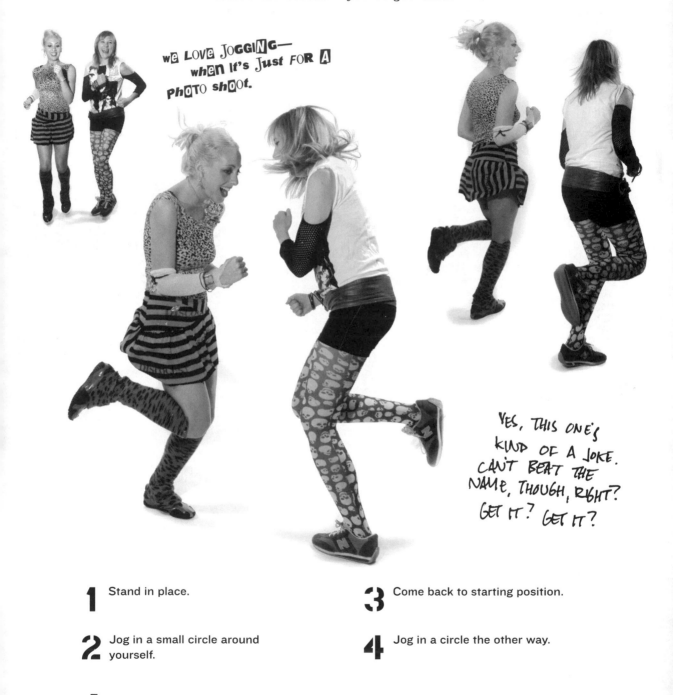

We love jogging— when it's just for a photo shoot.

Yes, this one's kind of a joke. Can't beat the name, though, right? Get it? Get it?

1 Stand in place.

2 Jog in a small circle around yourself.

3 Come back to starting position.

4 Jog in a circle the other way.

DEE DEE'S LUNGE

lo-fi / LEVEL: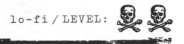

ALL YOU METAL KIDS are free to do this to Dee Snyder, but we had a certain Ramone in mind.

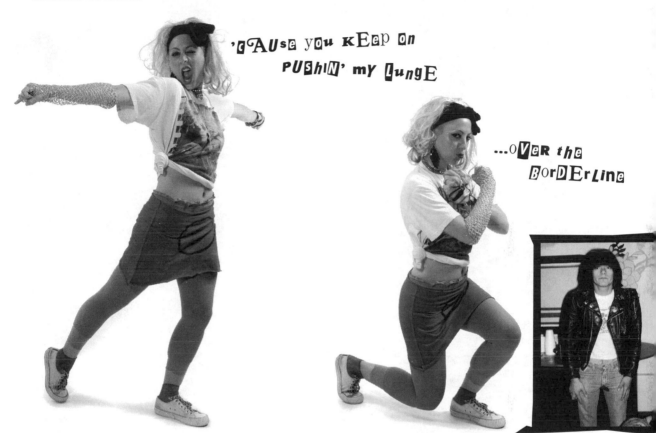

'CAUSe yOu kEEp On PUShiN' mY LungE

...OVeR tHe BorDErLine

Dee Dee Ramone

1 Stand facing straight ahead.

Turn to your left, bringing your right leg back.

Bring your arms to your sides, but not above your shoulders.

Make fists with your hands.

2 Bend both of your legs into the lunge position. Your back knee should almost touch the floor.

At the same time, lower your arms and cross them over your chest.

Come back up and bring the arms back to the starting position.

Turn and repeat on the other side.

* THIS IS BOTH LO-FI CARDIO AND STRENGTHENING;

WE THROW IT IN THE MIDDLE OF THIS SECTION TO LET YOU CATCH YOUR BREATH.

GREASED LIGHTNING hi OR lo-fi / LEVEL: ☠☠

YOU REMEMBER GREASE. Don't be so above it all.

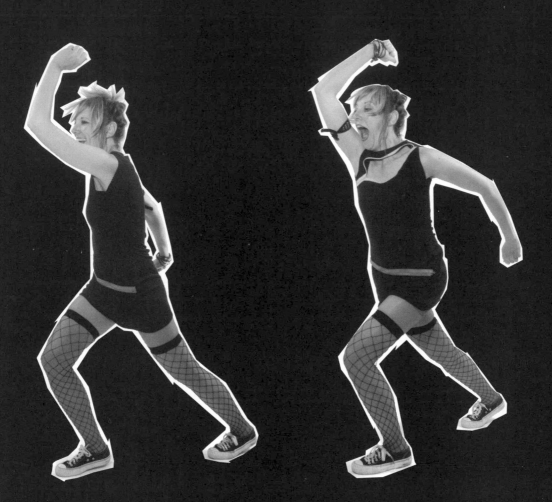

1 Stand in the lunge position with the right knee bent over your right foot, and the left leg straight back.

2 Go-Go your arms up and down, jump, and exchange your feet with your arms (as the right arm goes up, bring your left leg to the front).

→ MAURA'S BEEN WAITING FOR THIS EVER SINCE SHE GOT SHAFTED FOR THE ROLE OF RIZZO IN HER HIGH SCHOOL'S PRODUCTION OF GREASE.

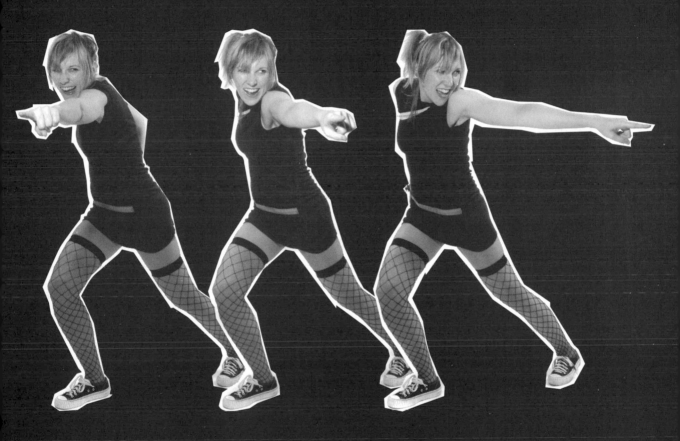

3 After you jump four times, stop and bring your arm straight out in front of you, Greased Lightning style.

4 When you've drawn a half circle around your body with your arm, jump and repeat the arm movement on the other side.

HAM CURLS

NO, this isn't a newfangled snack food.

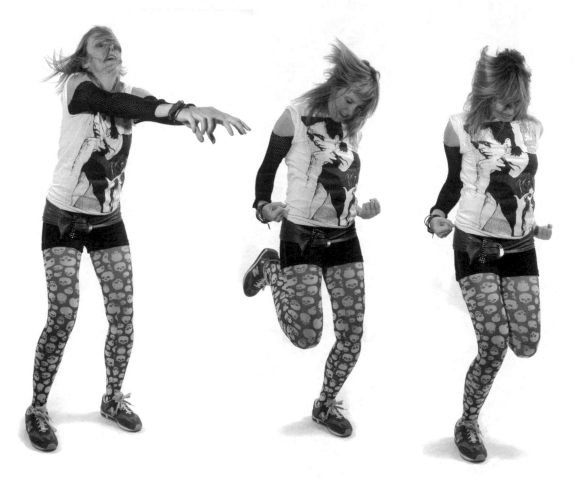

1 Start with your feet shoulder-width apart.

2 Shift your weight from side to side, bending your knees and bringing each leg up as you go.

Bring your arms in and out at the sides as you bend your legs.

3 Throw in a little hop as the arms come in and make it Hi-Fi!

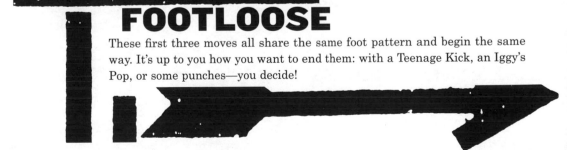

FOOTLOOSE

These first three moves all share the same foot pattern and begin the same way. It's up to you how you want to end them: with a Teenage Kick, an Iggy's Pop, or some punches—you decide!

TEENAGE KICK

hi OR lo-fi / LEVEL: ☠ ☠

THIS MOVE WAS INSPIRED by the song "Teenage Kicks" by the Undertones. We modeled a lot of moves on this one, so try to master it and the others will be a breeze.

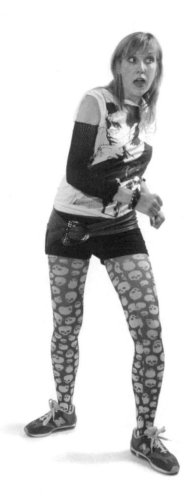 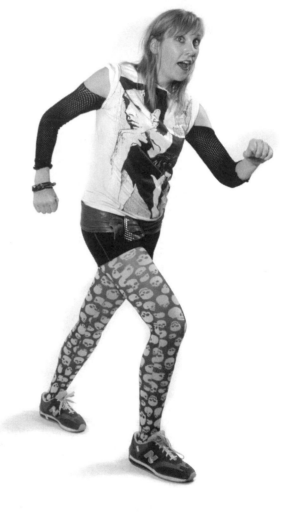

1 Stand facing straight ahead. Step out and to the left on a diagonal.

2 Step forward with your right foot.

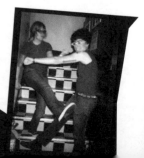

Erase Errata doing the Teenage Kick.

→ IF YOU WANT TO DO IT HI-FI, TRY A LITTLE JUMP OFF THE FLOOR EACH TIME YOU KICK AND PUNCH. IN CLASS WE SCREAM "STEP, STEP, KICK STEP, STEP, KICK!" AS WE DO THE MOVE. GIVE IT A TRY, UNLESS YOU HAVE NEIGHBORS WHO ARE EASILY PROVOKED.

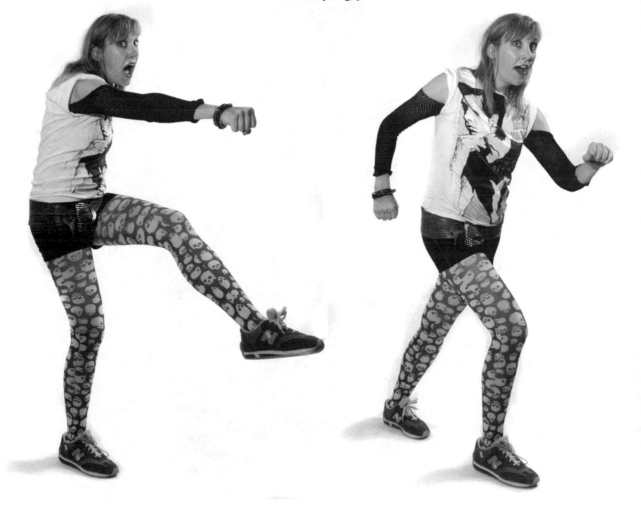

3 Kick out with your left foot; as you kick, punch with the opposite arm.

4 Step backward onto your left foot.

Repeat the pattern, turning to your right diagonal.

TEENAGE SKANK

hi OR lo-fi / LEVEL: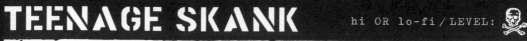

THIS MOVE is just like the Teenage Kick—but you end it with a skank instead!

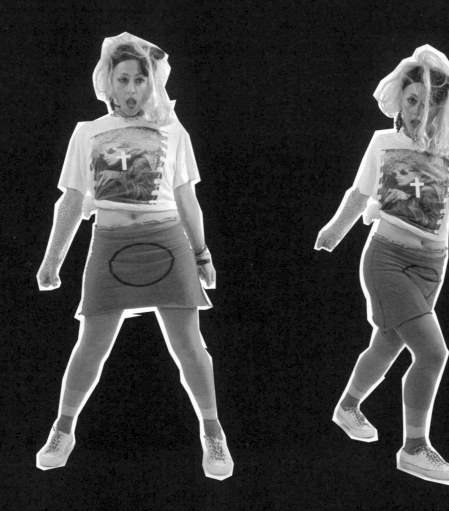

1 Stand facing straight ahead. Step out and to the left on a diagonal.

2 Step forward with your right foot.

* JUST LIKE THE TEENAGE KICK, YOU CAN DO THIS LO-FI OR HI-FI. TRY A LITTLE JUMP OFF THE FLOOR EACH TIME YOU SKANK TO HI-FI IT.

3 Skank, bringing the left leg up and throwing in an aggressive swing of the arms.

4 Step backward onto your left foot.

Repeat the pattern, turning to your right diagonal.

IGGY'S POP

YOU KNEW IT WAS COMING—we had to name something after him, even though some of Iggy's best moves involved rolling in peanut butter and broken glass then leaping headfirst into the crowd. Use his example as raw inspiration and go nuts.

*Don't F**K WiTh me, Jesus Is My homeBoy.*

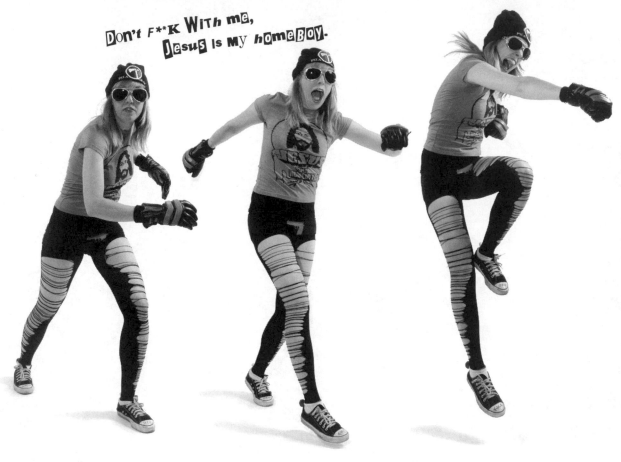

1 Stand facing straight ahead. Step to the diagonal with your left foot.

2 Step across with your right foot.

3 Raise the left knee waist high, and punch out with the right arm.

4 As you punch, throw in a jump.

Step backward onto your left foot.

IGGY'S PUNCH

FOR THE MANIMAL IN ALL OF US. When one punch isn't enough, try this and lose control! We recommend this for all of your favorite hardcore songs—the faster, the better.

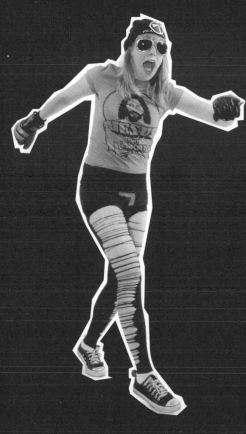

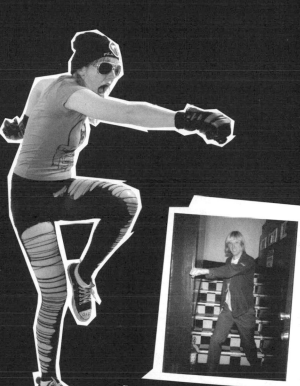

Eric Erlandson, from Hole, bustin' out his punch!

1 Repeat moves 1-3 of Iggy's Pop.

Step forward with your left foot, raise the right knee about waist high, and punch out with your left arm.

* THE MORE YOU PUNCH THE HARDER THE MOVE BECOMES. BETWEEN FIVE AND TEN PUNCHES IS GOOD; TRY TO FIND SOMETHING THAT FITS YOUR SONG.

2 Stay in place and repeat this punching motion. Punch out with your left arm, lifting and returning with your right leg.

Do five or more in succession, then switch to your other side and repeat.

Do this as many times as you want.

THIN THIGHS

THIS IS A PRA MODIFICATION of an exercise Hilken's mom used to do in her bedroom. She would refer to it as the "Thin Thighs."

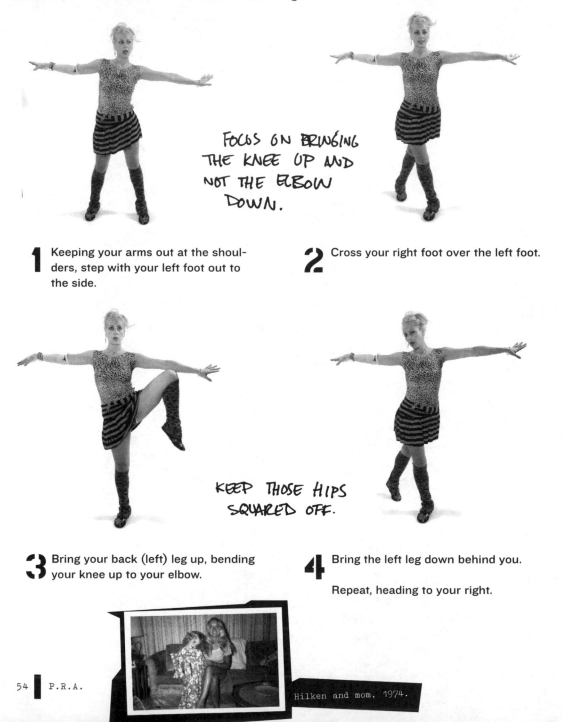

FOCUS ON BRINGING THE KNEE UP AND NOT THE ELBOW DOWN.

1 Keeping your arms out at the shoulders, step with your left foot out to the side.

2 Cross your right foot over the left foot.

KEEP THOSE HIPS SQUARED OFF.

3 Bring your back (left) leg up, bending your knee up to your elbow.

4 Bring the left leg down behind you.

Repeat, heading to your right.

54 | P.R.A.

Hilken and mom, 1974.

HIP SLUG

hi OR lo-fi / LEVEL: ☠ ☠

WE LIKE THIS MOVE cause you can make it as macho and sleazy as you like...with a little more frontal thrust it can be a real head-turner.

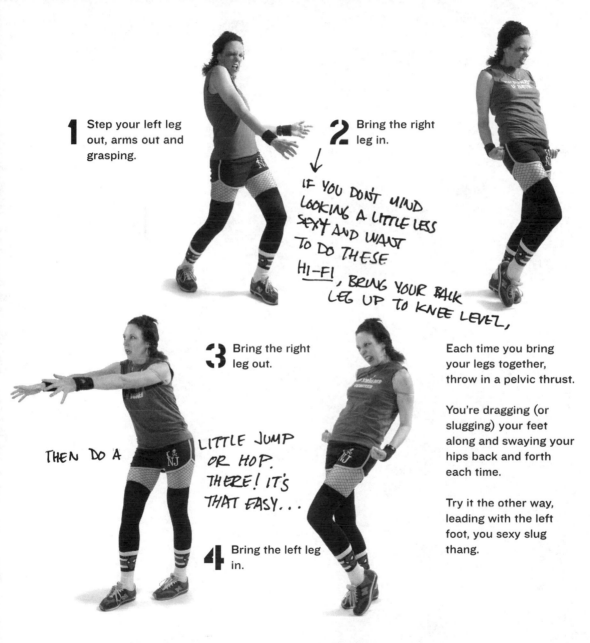

1 Step your left leg out, arms out and grasping.

2 Bring the right leg in.

IF YOU DON'T MIND LOOKING A LITTLE LESS SEXY AND WANT TO DO THESE HI-FI, BRING YOUR BACK LEG UP TO KNEE LEVEL,

3 Bring the right leg out.

THEN DO A LITTLE JUMP OR HOP. THERE! IT'S THAT EASY...

4 Bring the left leg in.

Each time you bring your legs together, throw in a pelvic thrust.

You're dragging (or slugging) your feet along and swaying your hips back and forth each time.

Try it the other way, leading with the left foot, you sexy slug thang.

...TO BE A HIP SLUG.

ROADRUNNER

lo-fi / LEVEL: 💀 💀 💀

IN CASE YOU WERE WONDERING, we invented this move to complement Jonathan Richman's song "Roadrunner." There are many versions, but our favorite is from the record called simply **THE MODERN LOVERS.** He sings about being in love with Massachusetts and driving around with the radio on. (We often wonder what station he was listening to, being Massachusetts gals.)

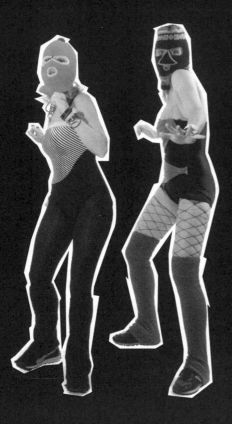

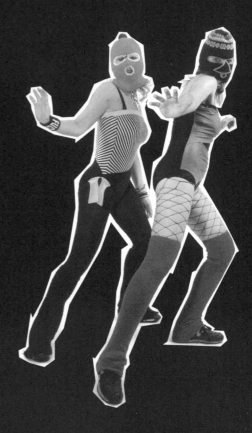

1 Start facing to the side. Bring your arms up to your sides, no higher than your shoulders.

2 Turn and make a half circle with your arm, so that you are facing the other side of the room.

* AS YOU SWITCH SIDES, THINK STEP, STEP, STEP, CLAP!

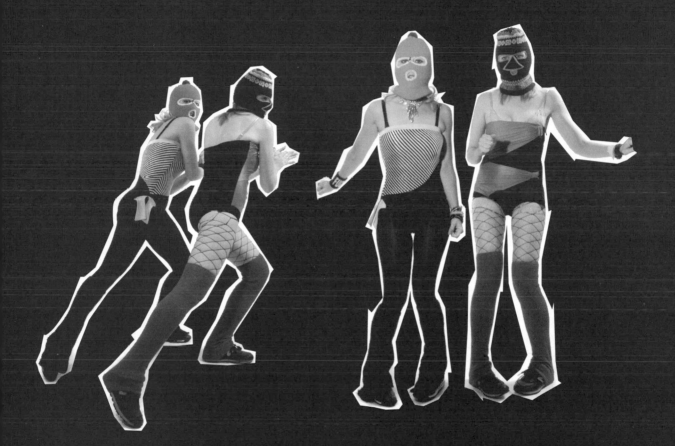

3 Clap your hands.

4 Bring your arms back to your sides and make a half circle to bring you back to the starting position.

Make half circles back and forth, clapping in between.

TRANSIENT SQUATTER

lo-fi / LEVEL: ☠ ☠ ☠

IT'S LIKE THE SQUATTER but it moves—for those of you who can't settle down.

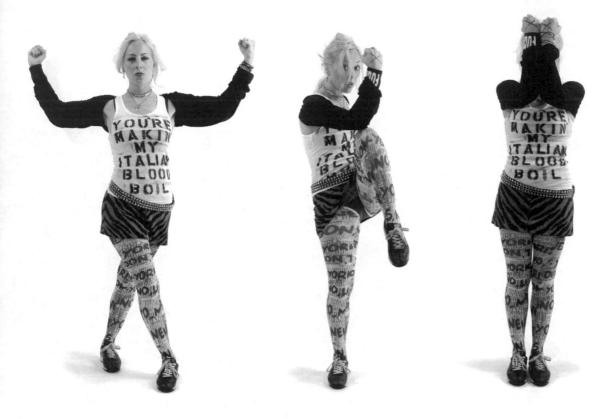

1 Cross your right foot over the left one.

Make an L shape with your arms.

2 Bring your left knee up to your right elbow.

Step back on the left leg, opening the arms back out.

3 Come into the center, bringing your arms in front of your face.

Now cross your left foot over and open the arms back out in a U shape.

Repeat the pattern, bringing your right knee up to your left elbow.

* SINCE YOUR ARMS ARE RAISED, IT FEELS A LOT TOUGHER TO MAINTAIN THAN SOME OF THE OTHER FOOTLOOSE MOVES. IT HELPS TO CHANT "STEP, KNEE, STEP, BACK."

DRISCOLL

WE NAMED THIS MOVE after our friend, Kristen Driscoll. It goes great to Blondie's "Heart of Glass," and once you've got it down, you'll feel like you're working the room at Studio 54. We usually throw this one in to give you a chance to catch your breath...so do it Lo-Fi most of the time.

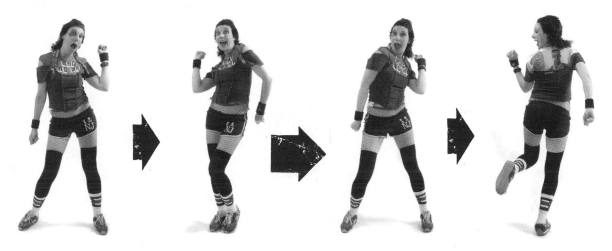

1 Stand facing straight ahead.

Step your left foot out to the side.

2 Bring your right foot in next to it.

3 Step to the side with your left foot again, but as you step, this time do a half turn to your left.

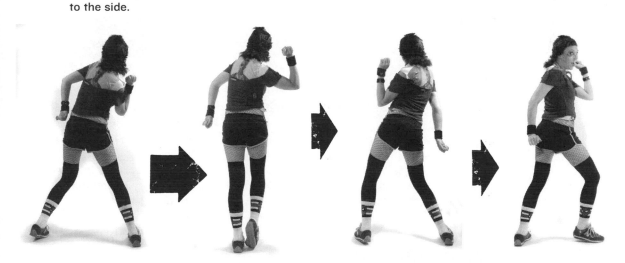

4 Now you'll be facing the back of the room: repeat, heading in the same direction starting with your right foot.

*IF YOU WANT TO DO IT HI-FI, TRY A LITTLE JUMP OFF THE FLOOR EACH TIME YOU TURN. ITS LESS DISCO, AND YOUR HEART WILL BE PUMPING MORE.

SWIZZLE-SWISH

IT MIGHT SOUND A BIT GIRLY to some of you macho men, but if you're secure about your sexual orientation, it's **FABULOUS**.

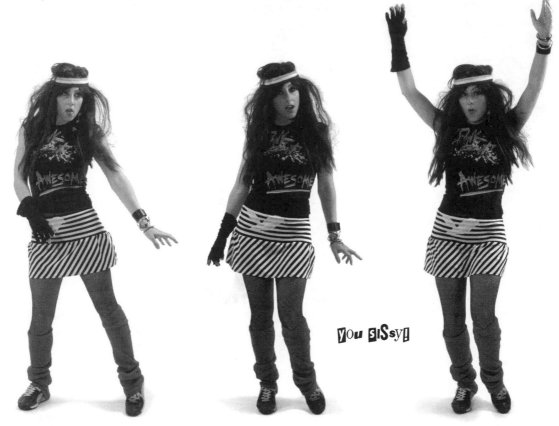

YOU SISSY!

1 Step your right foot out to the side.

2 Slide your left foot next to it, with a little hop, if possible.

3 Step your right foot out again, and slide your left foot in.

4 Swing your arms in a full circle around you, if you want.

Reverse direction, exchanging your left foot with the right.

→ JUST "SASHAY" FROM SIDE TO SIDE.

SWIZZLE-KICKS

 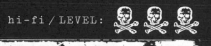

THIS IS LIKE THE SWIZZLE-SWISH, except at the end you do two punches.

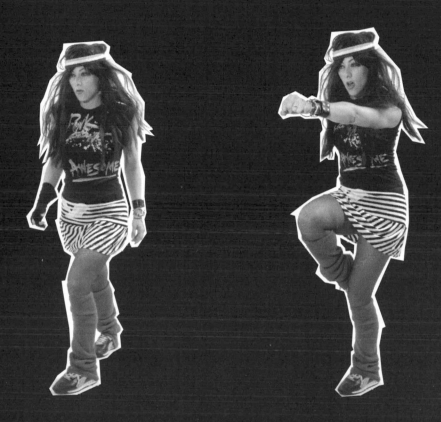

1 After steps 1-4 on the previous page, cross the left foot in front of the right.

2 Bring up your right leg to the knee and punch two times simultaneously.

Repeat this move in the opposite direction, exchanging your left foot with the right.

● THIS IS A COMBINATION OF SWIZZLE-SWISH AND IGGY'S POP PUNCH, ONLY TRY TO MAKE IT ONE SEAMLESS MOVEMENT. DON'T WORRY IF YOU ARE FUMBLING THROUGH IT. IT'S TOUGH TO MASTER, BUT FUN ONCE YOU GET THE HANG OF IT.

RUT DANCE

THIS IS A COMBINATION of two moves in one, but we liked it so much that we gave it its own name. Like Swizzle Kicks, it incorporates Iggy's Punch then throws a traditional aerobics V-step into the middle of it.

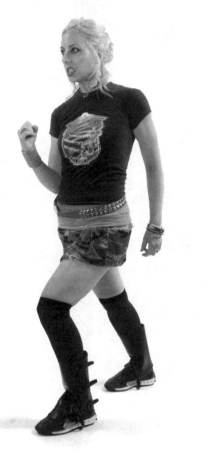
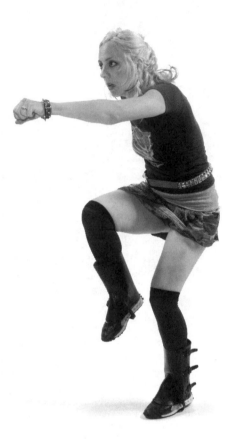

1 Step forward with your left foot. Now raise your right knee and punch out with the left arm.

2 Stay in place and repeat this punching motion three times.

You are punching out with your left arm, and lifting and returning with the right leg.

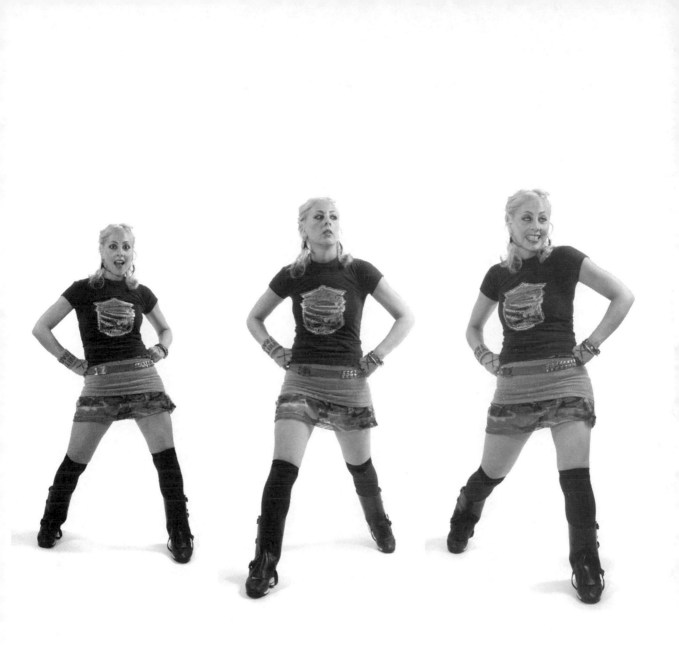

3 After your third punch, step back onto the right leg then onto the left, centering yourself and placing your weight evenly on both feet.

4 Step out onto your right foot and then your left, making a V with your legs twice (out and in, out and in).

Switch to your right side and **repeat**, raising your left knee.

THUG

THIS MOVE has some of the Swizzle Swish characteristics, but it's way more manly.

AMA LOOKS LIKE SHE'LL KICK YOUR ASS— AND SHE CAN.

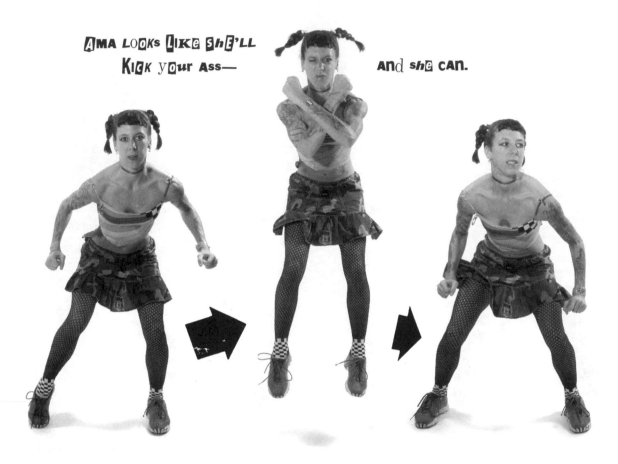

1 Step your left foot out to the side.

2 Slide and skip in your right foot.

Push off the floor, and as you do, cross the arms in front of you, both feet off the floor.

3 Step to the side onto your left foot.

Touch the ball of your left foot to the floor next to your right foot. Push and jump off the floor in the other direction, again crossing your arms.

Go back and forth from left foot to right.

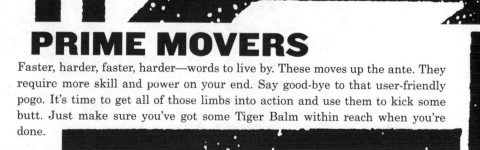

PRIME MOVERS

Faster, harder, faster, harder—words to live by. These moves up the ante. They require more skill and power on your end. Say good-bye to that user-friendly pogo. It's time to get all of those limbs into action and use them to kick some butt. Just make sure you've got some Tiger Balm within reach when you're done.

YOU BE THE STAR
AIR GUITAR

THIS IS THE CHANCE that we know you've been waiting for. It's time to find your inner guitar god and break out the licks. We like to throw in "windmills" a la Pete Townsend for added cardio kick, but you may have a favorite shredder move of your own. After all, personal style is the key to a winning air guitar.

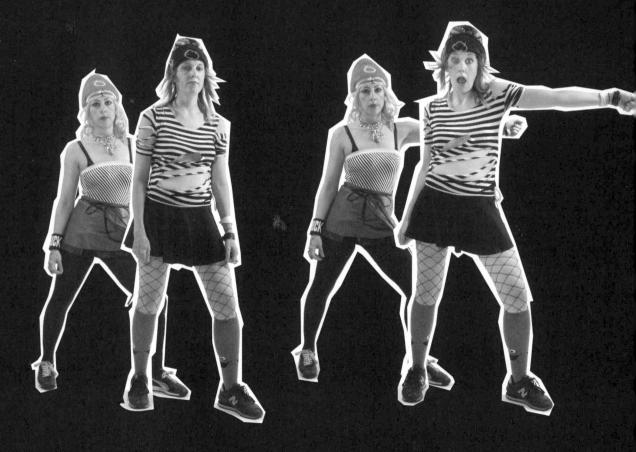

1 Stand in the lunge position with your left knee bent over the toe, the right leg back straight.

2 Bring your left arm straight out at your side (as if you were holding a guitar).

* WE JUMP TO A COUNT OF FOUR, BUT IF ANOTHER COUNT WORKS BETTER WITH YOUR SONG, GO FOR IT!

3 Swing your right arm in a circle, making a windmill.

As you swing the arm, kick your right leg straight out with it.

4 Jump up and down on your left leg, for a count of four.

Turn to your right and do this on your right side.

SUPER LUNGE

HOW TO PRODUCE TOXIC SWEAT: stay up all night smoking and drinking. Rip into a bag of chips before passing out in bed with empty chip bag gently rising and falling on your stomach. Wake up four hours later to a pounding headache and a desperate need for coffee. Pick a tune and do the Super Lunge for at least two minutes. If you don't puke the poison out, you're guaranteed to sweat it out. You cannot lose.

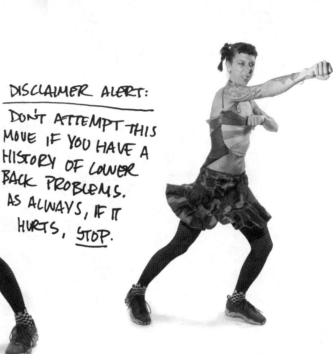

DISCLAIMER ALERT:

DON'T ATTEMPT THIS MOVE IF YOU HAVE A HISTORY OF LOWER BACK PROBLEMS. AS ALWAYS, IF IT HURTS, STOP.

1 Stand facing straight ahead. Jump and turn to the right, bringing your body into a lunging position as you land.

Your front leg should be bent (knee aligned over your toe), and your back leg extended straight behind you.

As you jump and turn to the right, punch out to the right with your left arm.

2 Try it on the other side.

Keeping the abs tight, punch the arms directly out from the chest area.

Keep the shoulders and hips in alignment as you jump and punch on each side.

Repeat in short bursts (ten seconds) or try for longer bursts of one to two minutes.

* USE CONTROLLED MOVEMENT. CONCENTRATE ON TURNING TO YOUR SIDE WITH EACH PUNCH, AND DO NOT SWING YOUR ARMS OUT RECKLESSLY OR USE JERKY MOVEMENTS.

ROTO-ROOTER

hi-fi / LEVEL: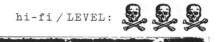

THIS IS A NEW BREED OF LUNGING EXERCISE. We came up with this move all by ourselves, and like all proud parents, we like to see our baby kick ass. Rest assured, it does.

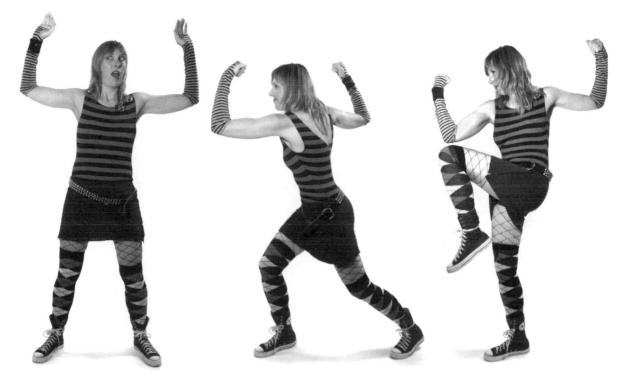

1 Stand facing straight ahead, feet shoulder-width apart, arms at your sides making an L shape.

Your hands are over your head, criminal style. Think, "No officer, I'm not armed," as Maura is thinking here.

YOU SHOULD NOT DO THIS MOVE TO A REALLY FAST SONG.

2 Jump and turn to the right, bringing your body into the lunge position as you land. (Same move as Super Lunge.)

3 Raise your left knee and bring your right elbow and left knee toward each other as if they were about to touch. (Don't worry if they don't touch, just give it your best shot.)

4 Bring your leg back down to its original position.

Keeping your arms raised the whole time, turn to the left and repeat.

Do this as many times as you want to.

SLITS LEG LIFTS

WE COULD GO ON AND ON about how cool the Slits were, but why bother? If you haven't heard them, run out and get a copy of **CUT**. The album cover shows Ari Up, Palmolive, Viv Albertine, and Tess Pollitt in the wild, naked and covered in mud, like members of a lost Amazonian tribe ready to devour an unfortunate anthropologist.

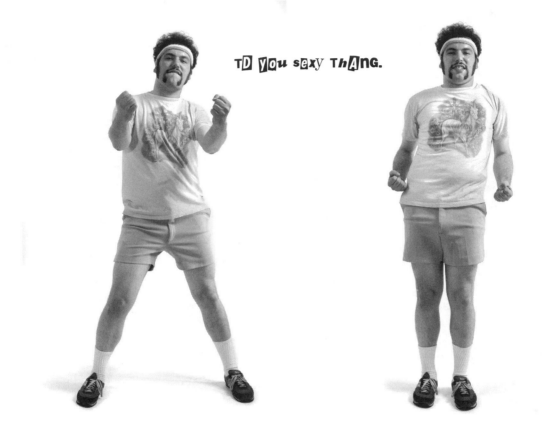

TO YOU SEXY THANG.

1 Stand facing straight ahead and step out to the side, arms straight out in front of you.

2 Raise the other foot and step in next to the leading one.

Bend your arms in at the hip.

→ REMEMBER: IT'S NOT THE SIZE, IT'S THE FLOW. WHO CARES HOW HIGH YOU GET THAT LEG TO LIFT? JUST KEEP IT GOING BACK AND FORTH. IT'S THAT EASY.

COME TO DADDY.

OOH, YEAH...

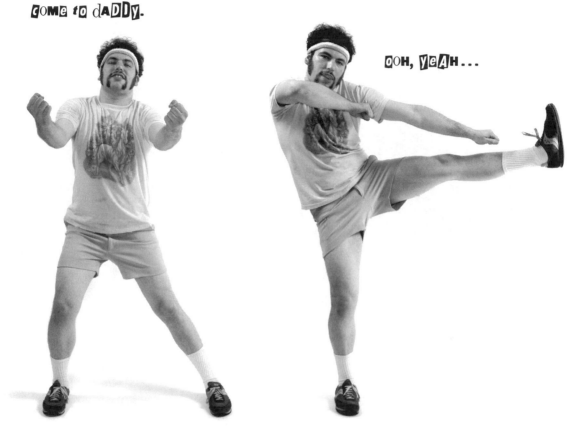

3 Step out again, and this time lift your other leg up into a side leg lift.

4 Swing the arms up to chest level, making a "bow and arrow." Lower your leg and bring the foot to the floor.

Follow and step in with the other foot.

Step out again and lift the other leg into a side leg lift with the opposite "bow and arrow" arms.

Keep this pattern going back and forth and flowing.

HEAD KICKED IN

WE CANNOT PROCEED without first mentioning that this move is possible only because of the Rezillos' bubblegum pop version of "Somebody's Gonna Get Their Head Kicked in Tonight"; fittingly, it is incredibly ridiculous. Find your meanest scowl for this one.

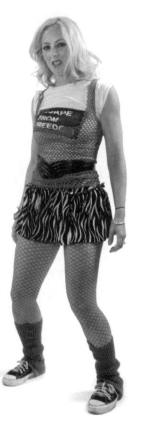

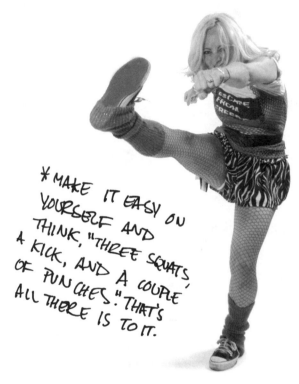

*MAKE IT EASY ON YOURSELF AND THINK, "THREE SQUATS, A KICK, AND A COUPLE OF PUNCHES." THAT'S ALL THERE IS TO IT.

1 Stand with your feet further than shoulder-width apart.

Your knees are slightly bent.

You are going to do three squats, or pliés, by bending the knees deeper than where they are now.

2 After the third bend, forcefully kick one leg out in front of you.

Punch out the arm opposite to the leg you kicked.

Return to starting position.

Repeat the three squats and then kick and punch with the other leg and arm.

P.R.A. Q&A #7

Hugo Burnham

Drummer for Gang of Four

....

When you think about getting into shape, does it make you think you have to radically change your lifestyle?

Yes, absolutely. I'm a fat f**k and I need to lose 60 lbs.

Did you ever get a doctor's note so you wouldn't have to take gym class?

No, I was always one of the first. Quite the sportsman, I was.

Do you have a gym membership?

Yes, at the Glouchester YMCA.

If you exercise, what type of exercise do you do? And what kind of music do you listen to when working out?

Unfortunately, the only real exercise I get is dancing with my three-year-old-daughter. We dance to 1) "Rock Lobster" by The B-52's (Daddy's song), 2) "Call Me Lightning," by The Who, 3) "Car Wash" by Rose Royce, 4) "Step in Time," and "The Chimney Sweep Song," from Mary Poppins, which is bloody exhausting, 5) "Pinball Wizard." You should see my daughter windmill. Old Uncle Pete would be proud.

Does Mike Watt's cycling regime make you want to go out and buy a bike?

Absolutely not. But I still read his e-mails.

Does Natalie Merchant's interpretive dancing inspire you?

Yes, to trip her up.

What are your thoughts on Danzig?

He has man-breasts.

Does Richard Simmons make you laugh or make you think of a scary clown?

Neither. He makes me think how f**king sad so many women must be to be so enamored of the little schmuck.

Have you ever pushed away the coffee table to dance 'til all hours of the morning?

Yes, but I just fell over drunk.

When you go on the road, do you lose weight or gain weight?

It's been 15 years since I was on the road, but all the booze and free food was evened out by the intense exercise of drumming as magnificently as I once did.

If you're on the road and one of your bandmates or fellow touring bands gets up to go for a jog, do you hate them or join them?

Excuse me, I was in an English rock band. What is jogging?

Has your state of being in shape ever affected your performance either positively or negatively?

I was in good shape back then, which was a lot easier, being in my twenties. My sweat was 60% Jack Daniels back then.

Is Frisbee a sport to you or just a major at Hampshire College?

See "jogging" above.

Do you like your body, or are you among the ranks of people who think that if they could just lose those ten pounds, they'd be perfect?

I am perfect. But I'd be a lot happier if I was 60 lbs. lighter.

As a performer in the public eye, has body image ever been a concern? Have you ever had outside pressure (that is, from a label, etc.) about your weight/shape?

EMI: Hugo, stop drinking.
HUGO: No!
EMI: Okay, then.

Is skinny better than buff?

Who cares?

Do you think that fat people get no respect?

A lack of respect has nothing to do with being fat. Only dumb people (like my mother-in-law) judge people by their body-type.

Are you afraid of dodgeball?

No. But it's a game for bullies.

JUMPIN' JACKED-UPS

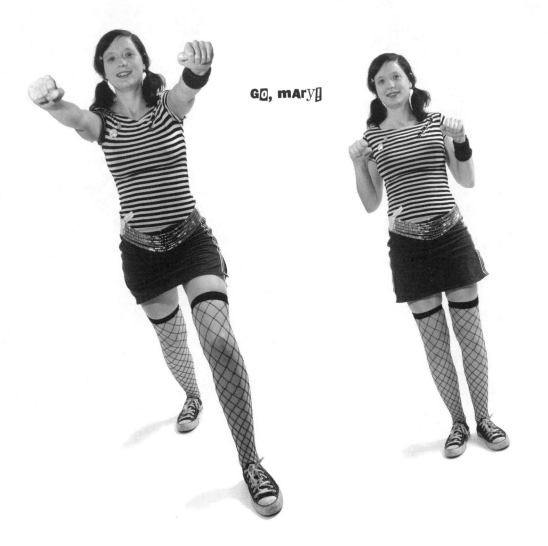

hi-fi / LEVEL: ☠ ☠

THIS IS A JUMPING JACK, jacked up **PRA** style.

GO, mAry!

1 Step backward onto your right foot, and reach with your arms straight in front of you, like a zombie.

Complete the move, stepping back with your left foot, and as you do, bring your arms in toward your body (as if rowing a boat).

IT HELPS TO CHANT:

"YOU GO BACK, YOU GO FORWARD, YOU DO TWO JUMPING JACKS—AGAIN!"

2 Step forward and reverse the move.

Do two jumping jacks.

Repeat.

SQUATTER

HOPEFULLY, you have no mirrors in the room where you are working out, 'cause this is one ugly move.

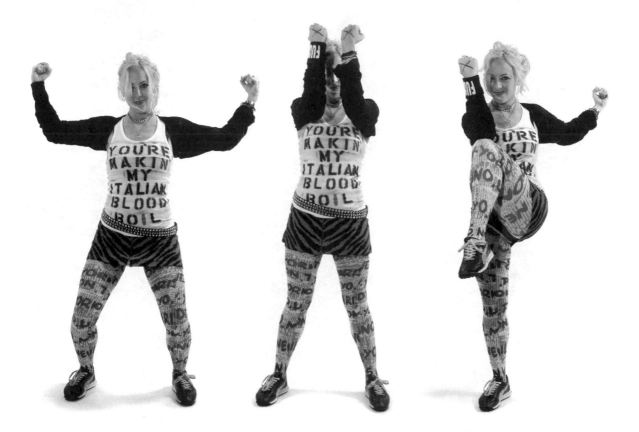

1 Stand facing straight ahead.

Make an L shape with your arms.

Bend your legs.

2 As you straighten your legs, bring your arms together in front of your face.

Bend your legs again and bring the arms back into position.

3 Straighten the legs and bring one knee up to the opposite elbow.

Repeat this pattern, bringing the other knee up to the opposite elbow, then switching back and forth.

*THIS MOVE IS ALOT LIKE ROTO-ROOTER — ONLY YOU DON'T MAKE IT ALL CRAZY AND HI-FI BY JUMPIN' AROUND.

PLUNGER

lo-fi / LEVEL: 💀 💀

THIS IS LO-FI BUT A TOTAL BALL BUSTER because your arms are up over your head practically the whole time. It's like the squatter, but with no bending of the knees in between.

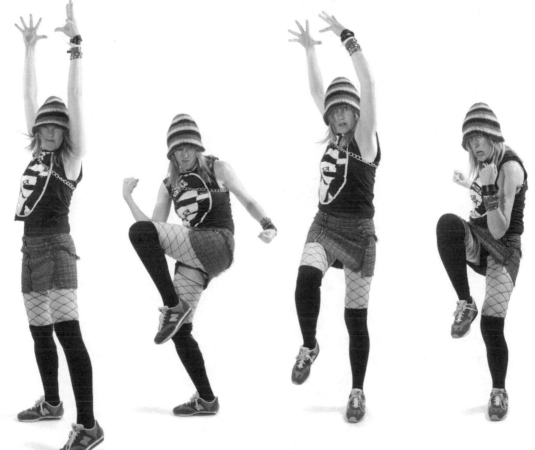

1 Raise your arms straight up over your head, making a straight line.

2 As you bring your arms down, bring your left knee to your right elbow. Bunch your hands into fists.

3 Raise your arms straight up over your head again.

4 Now bring them down and bring your right knee towards your left elbow.

Raise the arms up and bring them back down in this plunging type of move as the opposite knees and elbows meet.

PUNK ROCK COSMETICS

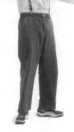

Inspired by Siouxsie Sioux

FROM GEEK TO FREAK, HERE'S OUR ART DIRECTOR, TRANSFORMED BY PUNK ROCK AEROBICS.

Fill in your eyebrow to make less of an arch. Use whatever eyebrow pencil or eyeliner looks to be the same color of your eyebrows

Get your blackest eyeliner and line the inner rims of your eyes (both upper and lower). Get *Clockwork Orange* with it and pull those eyelids up to get the black eyeliner in there all over. We know it makes your eyes run. Deal with it. Makeup is more important than your comfort and health.

Now put any frosty icy color you wish all over your eyelids. The icier the better. Think evil Snow White. Put it in the corners of your eyes and wing it out and up to your brow bone. Get messy and put some underneath your lower lashes too.

Now the moment of ingenuity you've been waiting for: get out a lighter (if you don't know any smokers, expand your horizons and meet some) and burn the tip of your black eyeliner with it. Burn it good.

Wait a couple seconds for it to cool off—don't be a moron—and then line only the outer half of your eye on both the upper and lower lash line.

Curl your eyelashes and put on tons and tons of black mascara. Do not under any circumstances wimp out with brown mascara.

Add a sandbox of white powder and some red goth lipstick. Alex is a manly man, so we used black here.

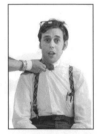
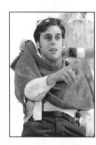
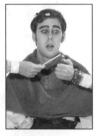
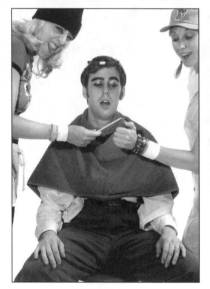
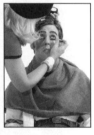
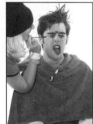
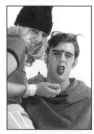
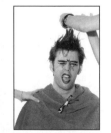

P.R.A. Q&A #8

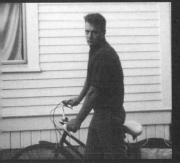

Calvin Johnson

Owner of K Records in Olympia, WA. Johnson was a member of Beat Happening, the Halo Benders and Dub Narcotic Sound System, and has performed as a solo artist.

Does Mike Watt's cycling regime make you want to go out and buy a bike?

Well ... I don't know anything about his bicycling regimen. However I have a great bicycle I got at Goodwill for only $12. It has a bell and a basket, and the basket is so great; you can take it off and use it to have a picnic.

Do you think William S. Burroughs ever lifted a weight in his life?

I know nothing about William S. Burroughs except that he lived in Lawrence, Kansas at the end of his life. I wanted to meet him, so when we were on tour there I knew he had all these shotgun paintings, and I figured it would be better to call and ask him if I could come by and check out these paintings, and he said yes, that sounded like a good idea. I had to leave 'cause we had a show in another town the next day, but he told me, "if you're ever in town again look me up."

Have you ever suffered an injury from improper instruction or insufficient knowledge about exercising?

I broke my finger playing football in sixth grade. Football doesn't make any sense to me. It's a dumb game. I think you can only like that game if you're an American who wants to conquer Third World countries.

Were you ever the last one to get picked for kickball in grade school?

That's me, yeah. Too short to get picked.

What kind of music do you listen to when working out?

None. It's best to concentrate fully on spacing out to whatever.

Does Richard Simmons make you laugh or make you think of a scary clown?

I saw the Howard Stern Show once, and Richard Simmons was on it. Howard Stern was giving him shit about being a homosexual, and Richard Simmons was being very kind and very gracious. Richard seemed like he was happy with who he was, and he seemed like a pretty cool dude. I'd wanna hang out with him.

Have you ever pushed away the coffee table to dance until all hours of the morning?

Oh Yeah. We do that all the time. I was just spinning records at The Dunes in Portland Oregon until about 5:00 a.m. Once when I was on tour and in Alfred, New York, I went to this party and there were 2 couches in the middle of this room that we were supposed to be having a dance party in, and I moved them into their hallway, one right on top of the other.

When you go on the road, do you lose weight or gain weight?

It probably depends on who the people on tour with me are. When you're on tour with people and they're like, "No ... we have to eat at all these wonderful restaurants all the time," then I do gain weight. But sometimes you're on the road with people and they're like, "I'll just a have a burrito."

Is Frisbee a sport to you or just a major at Hampshire College?

Frisbee makes no sense to me at all. It looks like it's coming at you and then it goes half a mile past you somewhere.

Has your state of "being in shape" ever affected your performance either positively or negatively?

Oh Yeah. Oh Man. There've definitely been times ... when I'm not quite there.

Have you ever had outside pressure (that is, from a label, etc.) about your weight/shape?

No. K is the only label. Every once in a while someone might say, "Hey Fatso"...I'll say, "Watch out. I will sit on you."

Are you afraid of dodgeball?

No, no. Slaughterball. I'd get out pretty early.

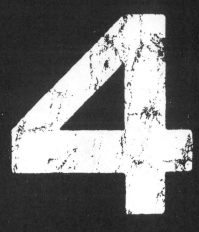

4

STRENGTH TRAINING

RAW

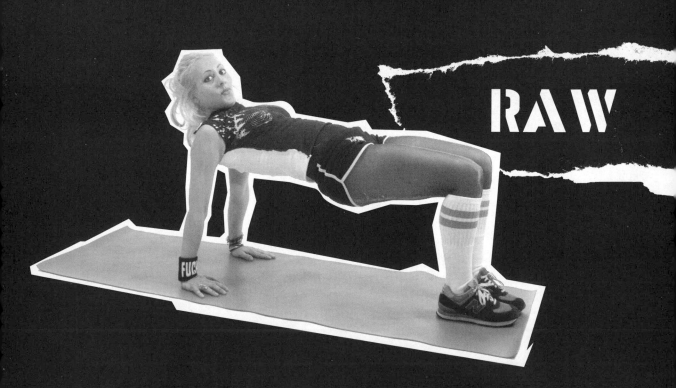

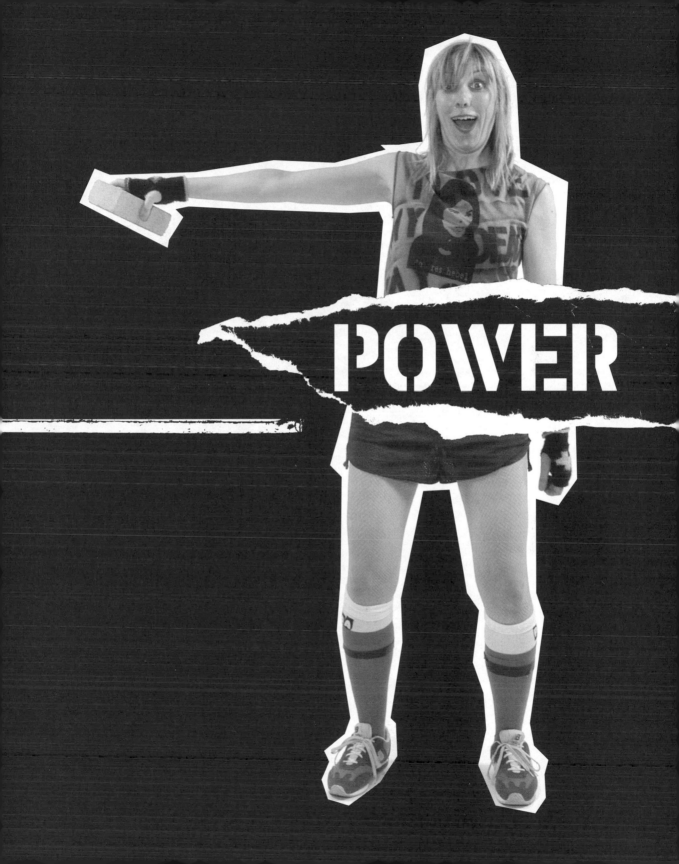

POWER

THERE'S A SCIENCE to the HOW of strength training. How often you do it, how fast you do it, what kind of training goes into it. Since we don't claim to be experts and most of you are just starting out, we're sticking to the basics.

BASIC TIPS FOR STRENGTH TRAINING

- DO EACH REPETITION SLOWLY AND WITH FOCUS. Blazing through your reps does nothing to help you. When it comes to strength training, slower is always better— don't rely on momentum to get the job done.

- PAY ATTENTION TO TECHNIQUE. When you perform and exercise incorrectly, muscles other than the one you are trying to exercise get into the act and help perform the task at hand. That's bad, because you don't build up the muscles you are trying to work.

- REMEMBER TO GIVE YOUR MUSCLES TIME TO REST AFTER WORKING OUT. Wait a day or two between strength-training sessions. They need time to rebuild so that they can become stronger the next time you attempt your workout.

- WORK EACH MUSCLE GROUP NO MORE THAN THREE TIMES A WEEK.

- INCREASE THE AMOUNT OF WEIGHT YOU USE SLOWLY, A LITTLE AT A TIME. If you aren't struggling through your last rep, then it is time for more weight.

SO NOW YOU CAN cardio train most of your chub into submission, but you've got to do more. Don't you want to be strong? By incorporating strength training into your three-move PRA combo-hatching, you'll become stronger and leaner, and develop better muscle definition. The following section includes a series of exercises to help you morph into a PRA terminator by addressing abs, ass, and arms. Wipe that look off your face. Sure it sounds like infomercial speak, but it works. We will explain how each of the muscle-building exercises is performed and how you can combine them to build a complete workout—but beware, these exercises really can improve your self-esteem. As your muscles expand, your ego might too. All things in moderation, as they say, for this is the stuff that transformed Charles Atlas and Henry Rollins from cowering nerds to empowered megalomaniacs....

To work out in front of a mirror and watch your body turn into a lethal weapon before your very eyes, start here. Cardio work strengthens your heart and pumps more power into your lungs, but these changes are invisible. Okay, it will also help you burn some fat, but without strength training it's going to take a *lonnnng* time before you see dramatic change. Strength training is all about muscle, and muscle is everywhere on the surface of your body. It's the single most important thing you can do to alter your physique. Did you know that each pound of muscle burns an extra thirty-five to fifty calories a day? This means that more muscle makes for a higher resting metabolism. Translation: you will be burning calories faster even if you are sitting on your pumped little ass reading the latest issue of *Jane* or *Mojo*. Strength training is also essential to maintaining a healthy, dense bone structure, which is an important weapon in the fight against osteoporosis. It is also instrumental in the prevention of arthritis, and in lowering the risk of cardiovascular disease. As you build strength, you replace fat with muscle. Fat is shapeless and makes your body look like a calzone with extra cheese. Muscle is dense and firm. It takes up less space, but also weighs more. This means that as you become stronger, you will lose inches, but you may gain weight. So look in the mirror and not at a scale. And don't worry about hulking out for the time being. You have to work your way up gradually. We know you are a long way off from shotputting a Jeep.

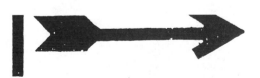

WE RECOMMEND STARTING WITH TWO - TO THREE - POUND WEIGHTS FOR WOMEN AND THREE - TO FIVE - POUND WEIGHTS FOR MEN. WORK YOUR WAY UP TO FIVE - TO EIGHT - POUND WEIGHTS AS YOU GET STRONGER.

GEtTiN' RIPPeD
ARMS and UPPER BODY

GETTIN' RIPPED means more than lifting a few pints from the bar to your mouth. You've got to start lifting if you want to rid yourself of that sunken chest and upper-arm flab. For each of the following exercises, you'll need to have a set of weights, even if those weights are bricks or two-liter soda bottles (see Chapter 1). When you're done, you'll be able to impress your friends by returning to the bar and trading in that pint you're guzzling for a pitcher!

Do the exercises slowly and carefully, and stay focused on the muscles you are working.

PUSS-UPS

DELTOIDS/PECTORALS/BICEPS/TRAPEZIUS/RHOMBOIDS (Shoulders, Boobs, Front of Arm, Back of Arm, Upper Back)

Get on your hands and knees

Your arms are shoulder-width apart, hands flat on the floor, wrists under your shoulders.

Slowly position your knees so that your upper legs are perpendicular to your back.

Slowly lower yourself down, pushing through with the chest.

You should almost touch your nose to the floor without extending your neck.

Slowly push yourself back up, completely straightening your arms.

As you lift and lower your torso to the floor, think of it as one unit.

Keep your back straight and abs tight to maintain position.

Your hips and shoulders should stay in alignment.

Do twenty.

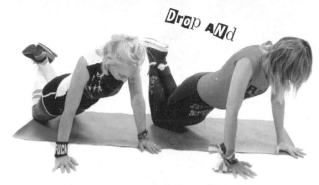

Drop aNd

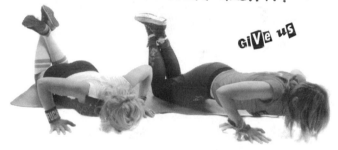

DON'T LET YOUR PELVIS SWAY OR YOUR BACK ARCH...

GiVe uS

...THIS WILL THROW YOU OFF BALANCE AND LESSEN THE EFFECT OF THE EXERCISE.

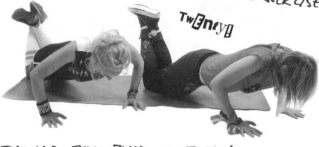

TwEnty

✱ TRY TO DO TEN, AND THEN BUILD TO TWENTY.

THIS IS A PUSH-UP, but we do it on our knees because we're pussies. It's harder than you think, so don't wuss out! For this exercise you will need a mat, or something else to cushion your knees.

BICEPTUAL

BICEPS (Front of the Upper Arm)

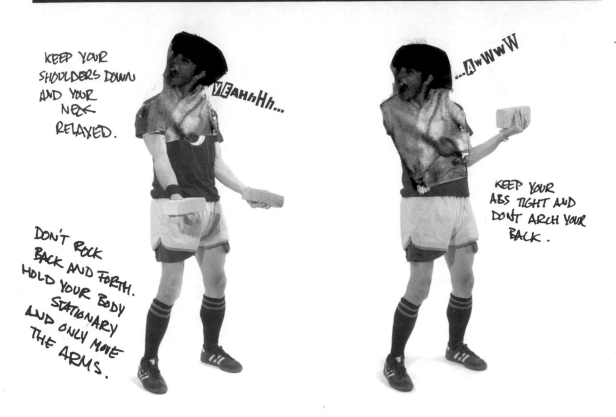

KEEP YOUR SHOULDERS DOWN AND YOUR NECK RELAXED.

YEAhhHh...

...AwwwW

KEEP YOUR ABS TIGHT AND DON'T ARCH YOUR BACK.

DON'T ROCK BACK AND FORTH. HOLD YOUR BODY STATIONARY AND ONLY MOVE THE ARMS.

Stand with your feet shoulder-width apart, knees slightly bent, a weight in each hand.

Slowly curl your forearms upward.

Your palms should be turned toward your shoulders.

Curl them up until you can't curl them any further.

Slowly lower back down.

Do twenty.

THIS IS A CLASSIC. When we do it in our class, we've got bricks in our hands and The Stooges blaring in the background. Do it enough times and people will be whispering that you might be biceptual. We outed **CLINT CONLEY** from Mission of Burma for this one!

SHOULDER-UPS

LEVEL: 💀 💀

DELTOIDS/TRAPEZIUS/PECTORALS (Shoulders, Upper Back, Boobs)

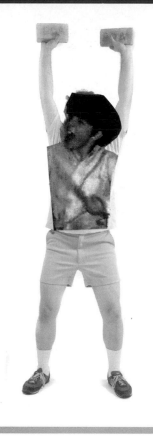

KEEP YOUR BACK STEADY AS YOU WORK.

Stand with your feet shoulder-width apart, your knees slightly bent.

Hold a weight in each hand at shoulder level.

→ DON'T ARCH YOUR BACK OR STICK OUT YOUR BUTT.

Bring your weights up until your arms are completely straight.

Do not snap the elbows or overextend the arms as you bring the weights up.

Slowly bring the arms back to the original position.

Do twenty.

THIS EXERCISE will help develop and define your entire shoulder. OWN THE PIT.

IRON MAN

DELTOIDS/TRAPEZIUS/PECTORALS/BICEPS (Shoulders, Upper Back, Boobs, Front of Upper Arm)

*DON'T LET YOUR ARMS DROP AS YOU GO BACK AND FORTH BETWEEN POSITIONS.

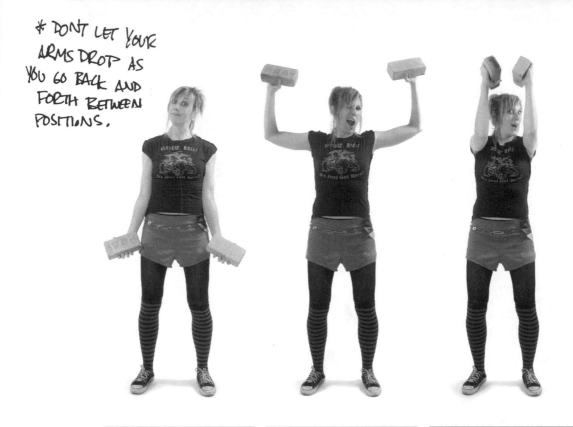

Stand with your feet shoulder-width apart, your knees slightly bent.

Hold a weight in each hand.

↓ TAKE A BREAK BETWEEN EACH SET OF TEN.

Bring your arms out to your sides and bend them into an L shape.

Holding your abs tight, move your arms toward each other, in front of your face.

Return your arms to their original L position.

Do twenty.

WHEN WE DO THIS IN CLASS there is a group moan that happens around rep number eight. We always laugh 'cause when it doesn't sound like a dying whale, it could almost be mistaken for "Ohm."

☆ REMEMBER TO SLOWLY RAISE THE ARM TO A STRAIGHT POSITION; DON'T SNAP THE ELBOW AND OVEREXTEND THE ARM.

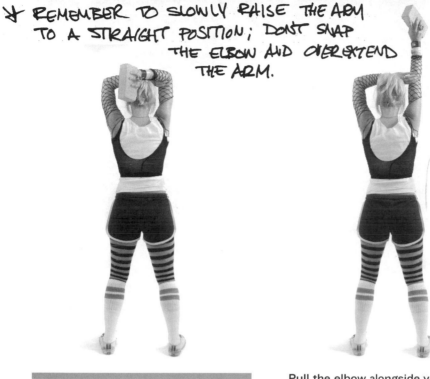

KEEP YOUR STOMACH SUCKED IN. MAKE SURE YOUR BACK IS NOT ARCHED AND YOUR TAILBONE IS POINTING DOWN TO THE FLOOR

Stand with your feet shoulder-width apart, your knees slightly bent.

Put a weight in one hand. Raise your arms above your head.

Bend the arm holding a weight behind your head.

With the other arm, reach over your head and grasp the elbow of the arm holding the weight.

Pull the elbow alongside your head, and keep it supported there throughout the exercise.

Raise the weight up above your head, then lower it back behind your head.

Do ten on each side, for a total of twenty repetitions.

WE HAVE TO CREDIT our fellow Punk Rock Aerobicizer T. D. Sidell for coming up with this name. PEEE-UUUUUU!

THE CHICKEN WING

LEVEL: ☠☠☠

TRICEPS (Back of Upper Arm)

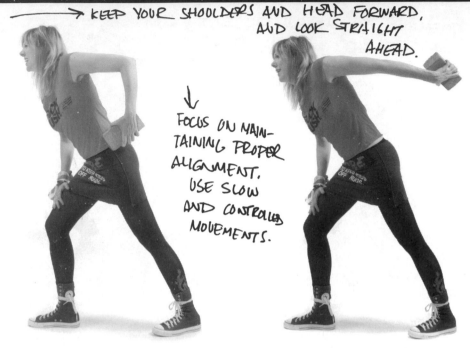

KEEP YOUR SHOULDERS AND HEAD FORWARD, AND LOOK STRAIGHT AHEAD.

FOCUS ON MAINTAINING PROPER ALIGNMENT. USE SLOW AND CONTROLLED MOVEMENTS.

Stand in the lunge position with the right knee bent over your toe, left leg straight back.

Align your back so that it forms a continuous straight line with your back leg. Imagine a plank running from the top of your head to the heel of your rear foot.

Hold a weight in one hand at your hip, palm facing your body.

Stretch the arm holding the weight straight behind you, as high as you can.

Slowly bend the elbow and return to starting position.

Never move the upper arm, and keep it at a 90-degree angle to the ground as you bring the weight back to your hip. Your arm should only move from the elbow down.

Do ten.

RID YOURSELF OF BINGO ARM, that wiggly-jiggly stuff that swings back and forth as you reach across the bar for that last can of PBR.

CHICKEN WING PART 2

LEVEL: ☠☠☠

TRICEPS (Back of the Arm)

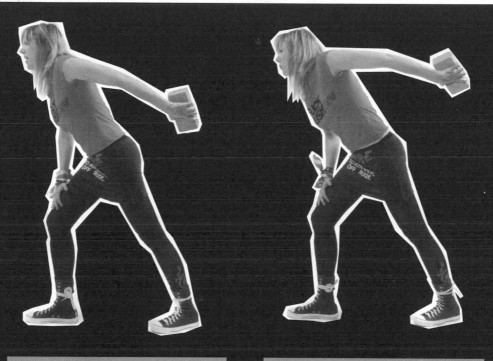

Stand in the same position you used in the Chicken Wing.

Your arm is extended behind you and in Chicken Wing position, holding a weight.

Your palm, holding the weight, is facing the ceiling.

Pulse up and lift your arm as high as you can.

Slowly lower your arm back to the starting position.

Do ten.

Now switch sides and do the entire Chicken Wing exercise on the opposite side.

* FOCUS ON YOUR MUSCLE. YOU SHOULD FEEL A BURNING AT THE BACK OF YOUR ARM, SO YOU KNOW IT'S WORKING.

AFTER YOU'VE REPEATED Part 1 ten times, flap right into Part 2.

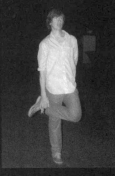

Thurston Moore

Singer and Guitarist for
Sonic Youth

....

Does Mike Watt's cycling regime make you want to go out and buy a bike?

Not since he got a hair inverted into his sweating crotch and nearly croaked from infection. Now he paddles in a kayak, which is way more punk. I gotta out-punk him and start hang-gliding.

When you think about getting into shape, does it make you think you have to radically change your lifestyle?

I'm 45, and my sunken chest and pear belly are not as charming as they may once have been. Kim gave me a gift certificate about three Christmases ago for a free pilates session. The time is nigh I'm ready to crunch. I have to. It's not really fair to Kim; she has a super-hot body and mine is a lumpen blob.

Were you ever the last one to get picked for kickball in grade school? Did you ever get a doctor's note so you wouldn't have to take gym class?

I was always last, and for some reason I used to always try and make sure that I was, as I knew that was my lot. It's weird because I also knew I could probably be a dodgeball dynamo, but alas, I was merely a meek dork.

Do you think William S. Burroughs ever lifted a weight in his life?

As a gay lover he must've lifted some kind of man-weight.

Have you ever suffered an injury from improper instruction or insufficient knowledge about exercising?

I have to be careful, as I have a lens implant in my right eye from a detached retina if I put the wrong kind of yoga pressure on it my eye will spurt and pop out of my face. Really, it's true.

If you exercise, what type of exercise do you do? And what kind of music do you listen to when working out?

I walk through the woods of Smith College in Northampton, Massachusetts, listening to recordings of Sylvia Plath. Again, really.

Does Richard Simmons make you laugh or make you think of a scary clown?

He makes me happy mostly, but not so much in a rock 'n' roll way.

When you go on the road, do you lose weight or gain weight?

We usually start our tours ripping through the South, and I start getting BBQ belly, but when we traverse the North and the West I begin to slim down with tofu, sushi and smoothies.

Is Frisbee a sport to you or just a major at Hampshire College?

It's kind of like squaresville hackysack in a way-both activities make me sad to be male.

If you're on the road and one of your bandmates or fellow touring bands gets up to go for a jog, do you hate them or join them?

This has not happened-it is forbidden. We only allow cerebral fitness programs, and even those can become annoying.

Has your state of "being in shape" ever affected your performance either positively or negatively? Do you tend to work up a sweat onstage?

It matters how many mommas are in attendance, re: sweat. I suppose if I were in decent shape like Bruce Springsteen I'd play all night long, but I've got a lot of other shit going on.

Do you like your body, or are you among the ranks of people who think that if they could just lose those ten pounds, they'd be perfect?

It's not so much the poundage as the roundage which I have a problem with. I like the way my body feels sometimes but I don't really dig the way it looks.

As a performer in the public eye, has body image ever been a concern? Have you ever had outside pressure (ie from a label) about your weight/shape?

No, in punk rock an ugly body has the validity to be hot.

QUADRUPED

LEVEL: ☠☠☠

PECTORALIS/TRICEPS/MINOR BICEPS/BRACHIALIS (Chest, Arms, Back of Arms)

Lie on the floor with your knees bent and arms by your sides.

Raise yourself up, palms face down, hands in a straight line underneath your shoulders, facing forward.

Squeeze your buttocks and raise your torso off the floor as one unit. You should look like a coffee table.

Now lower and lift your entire torso by bending and straightening only your arms.

Most of your weight should be on your arms, not on your feet.

Don't let your ass dip. Hold yourself up by squeezing your buttocks and make your ass tight as you lower it up and down.

Do ten.

Lay back down into your starting position, then do ten more.

HILKEN takes great pride in this one, so don't try to mess with her. It takes a lot of skill to be a human coffee table.

THE IGGY

TRICEPS/PECTORALS (Back of Arm, Boob Area)

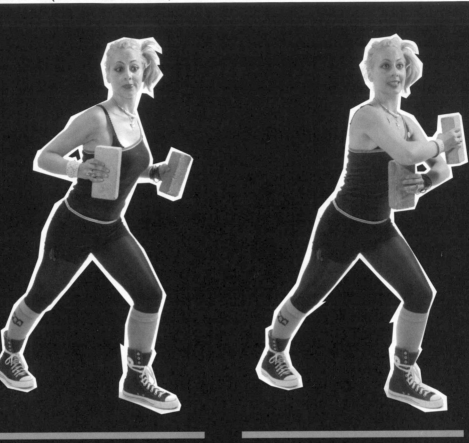

Stand in the lunge position with the left knee bent over your toe, right leg back straight.

Hold a weight in each hand.

Raise your arms up to stomach level with your elbows bent at your sides.

Cross your right arm over your left arm (Position 2).

Make sure you're crossing them directly in front of your stomach.

Bring arms back to step one.
Pulse back and forth ten times between steps one and two.

SUGGESTED LISTENING: The Stooges, "Search and Destroy." There simply is no other choice.

* WHEN RAISING YOUR ARMS TO THE ELEVATED AND CROSSED POSITION, DON'T BRING YOUR SHOULDERS UP WITH THEM.

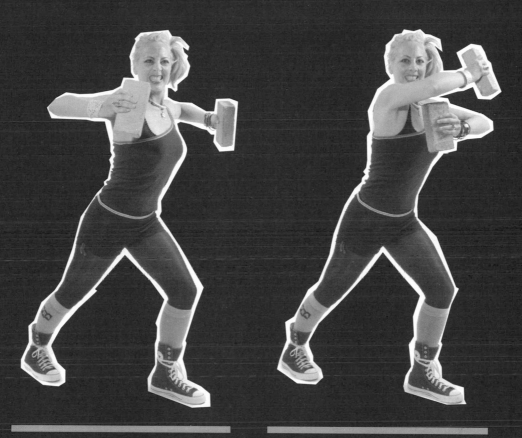

From there, slightly raise the arms upward in the crossed position. This time your arms are raised to breast level.

Pulse back and forth in the elevated position ten times.

Do ten.

Do this twice on each side, reversing the stance, with left arm above the right arm.

THE ARM OPPOSITE YOUR EXTENDED LEG IS THE ONE THAT'S CROSSING ABOVE. KEEP THEM RELAXED AND CONVERED. HOLD YOUR BACK STRAIGHT AND YOUR STOMACH IN.

BUTTERFLIES

DELTOIDS/PECTORALS (Shoulders & Boobs)

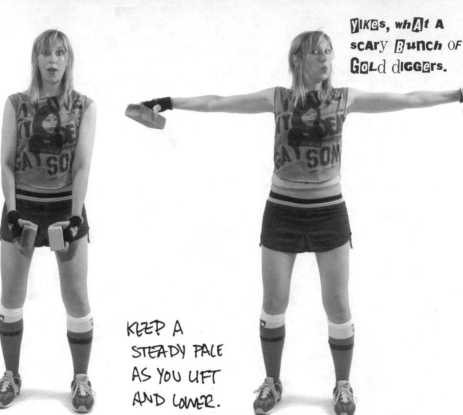

Yikes, whАt А scАry Bunch OF GoLd diGGers.

KEEP A STEADY PACE AS YOU LIFT AND LOWER.

Stand with your feet shoulder-width apart, your knees slightly bent.

Hold a weight in each hand.

Place your hands at your side with your palms facing each other.

Slowly raise your arms to your sides, no higher than your shoulders.

Slowly lower your arms back down to the starting position.

Do twenty.

MAURA was watching JOE MILLIONAIRE when these pictures were taken.

SUGGESTED LISTENING: "Repetition," by The Fall.

BUTTERFLIES PART 2

LEVEL: 💀 💀

DELTOIDS/PECTORALS (Shoulders & Boobs)

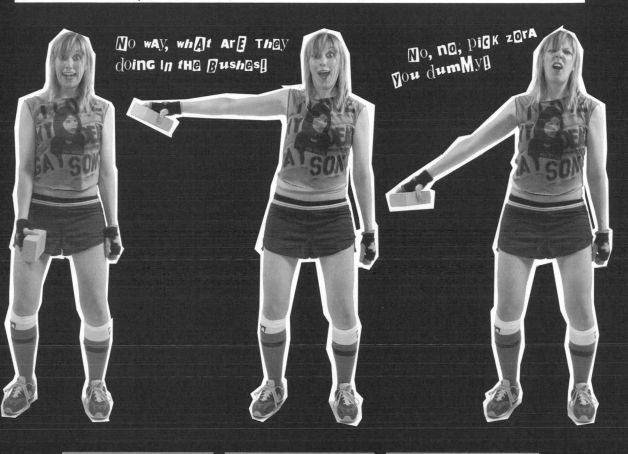

No wAy, whAt ArE thEy doIng In thE Bushes!

No, no, picK zOrA you dumMy!

Stand in the same position as in the previous exercise, a weight in one hand.

Raise your arm out to your side, with your palm facing down.

Raise your arm to shoulder height.

Pulse your arm up and down, lowering it about halfway to your hip.

Do five.

Repeat with your opposite arm.

Do ten, alternating arms right, left, right, left, and so on.

* TRY TO KEEP YOUR SHOULDERS RELAXED AND LOWERED. KEEP YOUR WEIGHT CENTERED AS YOU WORK. HOLD YOUR BODY STATIONARY AND ONLY MOVE THE ARMS.

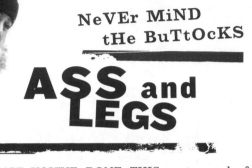

NeVEr MiND tHe BuTtOcKS

ASS and LEGS

ONCE YOU'VE DONE THIS next round of exercises, you'll know why we call them Rump Roasters. There are only four of them, but you must pay attention to technique if you want to reap the benefits. We suggest that you always do the Leg Lifter and combine it with two others. We like to listen to "Slang King" by The Fall. We get a kick out of the lyrics—if you listen closely you can hear Mark E. Smith say "Leg Lifter" over and over. And no, we're not high.

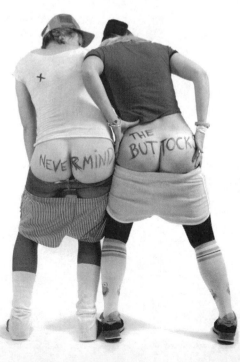

LEG LIFTER 1

LEVEL: ☠☠

Starting position:

Kneel down and bend forward, placing body weight on your elbows, hands clasped for additional support.

Your elbows should be shoulder-width apart, hips directly over your knees.

SMALLER MOVES ARE BETTER.

DON'T AIM FOR HEIGHT AND KICK THE LEG OUT TOO HIGH. YOU MAY END UP OVEREXTENDING, OR ARCHING YOUR BACK.

Set I

Bend your leg in toward your chest.

Extend and straighten your leg back behind you so that it's parallel to the mat.

Bring the leg back in to the chest.

Repeat, bringing the leg in and extending it back out.

Do ten

IF YOU ONLY HAVE TIME FOR ONE OF THESE EXERCISES, then this is the one you should do. Here's why: It works three large muscle groups, including the quads. The quads are the largest group of muscles in your body. The larger the muscle group the more work your body has to do, and the more calories you expend. Simple. TEN MINUTES spent working the quads is far more time efficient than ten minutes spent working one of your fingers. The LEG LIFTER gives you bang for your buck. It will leave your ass a burning cinder.

LEG LIFTER 2

 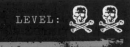

GLUTEUS MAXIMUS/QUADS/HAMSTRING (Leg & Ass)

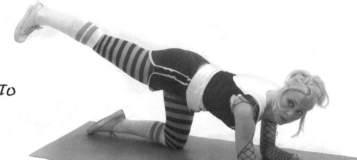

* BE CAREFUL NOT TO PULSE UP AND DOWN TOO HIGH OR TOO HARD.

YOUR UPPER BODY SHOULD REMAIN COMPLETELY STILL.

REMEMBER TO HOLD THOSE ABS TIGHT AND YOUR BACK STRAIGHT. ISOLATE THOSE BUTT MUSCLES.

Set 2

Keep the extended leg straight out.

Pulse the leg up and down, using small movements.

Do ten

* FOCUS ON ELONGATING THE MUSCLE HERE, AND STRETCHING YOUR LEG AS YOU STRAIGHTEN IT OUT.

Set 3

Keep the extended leg straight out.

Flexing the foot, bend the leg toward your back, forming an L shape with your leg.

Return your leg to the extended position, straight out and parallel to the mat.

Repeat, bending in and backing out.

Do ten

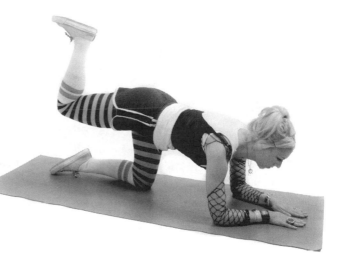

LEG LIFTER 4

LEVEL:

GLUTEUS MAXIMUS/QUADS/HAMSTRING (Leg & Ass)

* YOU SHOULD BE FOCUS-
ING ON YOUR BUTT
MUSCLES AND FEELING
THE PULSE. IMAGINE
THE SOLE OF YOUR
FOOT TOUCHING
THE CEILING.
→ APPLY CONTINUAL
TENSION TO YOUR WORKING
BUTT MUSCLE FROM THE
BEGINNING AND STARTING
POSITIONS. ~~____~~ YOU'LL
WANT TO SQUEAL LIKE A
PIG, BUT IT REALLY WORKS.

Set 4

Keep leg in L shape.

Pulse up and down.

Do ten

SLUT BUTT

LEVEL:

GLUTEUS MAXIMUS (Ass)

Lie on the floor with your knees bent and arms by your sides.

Feel as if you're pressing your upper back into the floor. Lift your pelvis up slowly.

Once your hips are elevated, squeeze your butt cheeks together.

Feel like you're keeping your spine straight the whole time you are doing this exercise.

Once you've raised and squeezed, slowly lower your ass back to the mat.

Do twenty

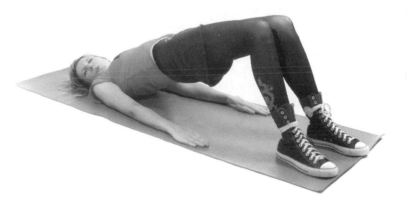

LIKE WE REALLY have to explain to you guys why we call it "Slut Butt." For a cheap laugh, do this one to Iggy Pop's "I Wanna Be Your Dog."

FIRE HYDRANTS

LEVEL: ☠ ☠ ☠

HIP ADDUCTORS/GLUTEUS MAXIMUS/QUADS (Thighs)

You are positioned on your hands and knees like a dog.

Bring your leg out to the side, keeping your knee bent.

Try to lift your leg out high enough to form a 90-degree angle. (Not all of us have great hip rotation but do your best, and lift your leg as high as you comfortably can.)

Extend and straighten your leg out to the side.

Bend your knee and bring your leg back into an "I'm peeing on a fire hydrant" position.

Now lower your bent leg back into its original starting position.

Do ten

Switch legs and repeat.

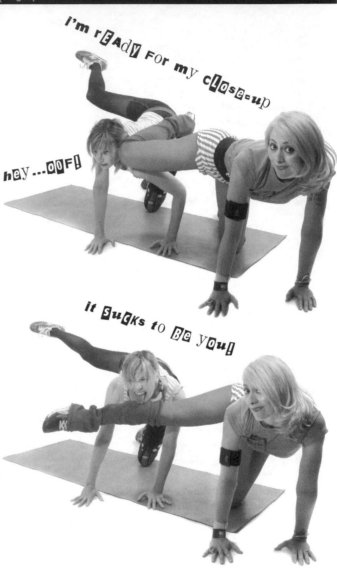

i'm rEAdy For my clOse-up

hEy...OOF!

it SuCks to Be you!

THIS ONE is oddly enjoyable when performed en masse—you look like an army of dogs drenching every hydrant in a two-block radius. It can also be rather difficult, Maura could only do four when we first started, so don't feel too bad; if your leg starts to shake and drop, just add on as you get stronger.

HYDRANT PLUS

LEVEL: ☠ ☠ ☠

HIP ADDUCTORS (Thighs)

nOW It SUCKs to BE ME!

Position yourself on hands and knees.

Keep your back straight and hands directly below your shoulders.

Extend your right leg straight out to the side so that it's perpendicular to the mat. Try to keep your left hip directly over the left knee.

Pulse the extended leg up and down.

Ten on each leg, for a total of twenty.

IF YOU STILL want to keep going after Fire Hydrants, then this is an easy one to add on. This is done in the same position and alignment as FIRE HYDRANTS, and if it's done right afterward, it can be a serious butt incinerator.

FACE DOWN BUTT LIFT

LEVEL: ☠☠

GLUTEUS MAXIMUS (Ass)

Lie down on your stomach, arms bent and forehead resting on your hands.

You are facedown, with your legs extended straight out behind you.

AM i Done yET?

Keeping your knees locked, lift one leg up off the ground and feel your butt muscle flex.

Hold for two seconds.

Do this without arching your back, and feel your hipbone press into the floor.

Slowly lower leg to the starting position.

Switch and repeat this exercise with your other leg.

Twenty times each.

*DON'T PUT THE PRESSURE ON YOUR LOWER BACK. FEEL THE WORKOUT IN YOUR BUTT MUSCLE ONLY.

i GOTtA GO Bid oN some EFFectS BOXEs On eBay.

MOST GUITAR GODS have strong arms, but their butts usually need extra work. We knew that this would be perfect for our friend J Mascis, who likes to spend a lot of time lying down.

THE MOVING UNIT

GLUTEUS MAXIMUS/HAMSTRINGS/SPINE EXTENSORS (Ass, Back of Legs)

Lie on the floor with your knees bent and arms by your sides.

Straighten out one leg so that it makes a 45-degree angle, and the knee is in line with the other knee.

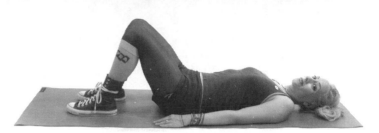

MAKE SURE YOU ARE PRESSING YOUR SHOULDERS AND UPPER BACK INTO THE FLOOR

Holding this position, squeeze your butt and hold your abs tight as you push and lift your hips off the floor, until your body forms one straight line from your toe to your shoulder to your hip.

Maintain the position and keep the leg level the entire time.

Slowly lower your torso back down as one unit to the mat.

Do ten.

Repeat and switch to your other leg.

YOU ARE MOVING UNITS, BABY!

IF YOU'VE EVER been dropped from your record label you'll know what it means if you don't move enough units.

Lie on your side, supporting yourself on your elbow, or lie down flat with your head resting on your arm.

Bend the leg you're not working and place the sole of that foot on the ground in front of you.

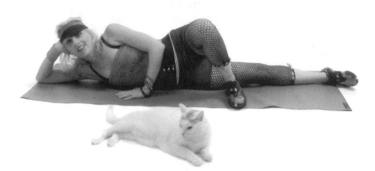

Lift the other leg slightly off the ground, until it can't go any higher.

Lower leg halfway down to floor.

Pulse up and down.

Do ten and switch legs for ten.

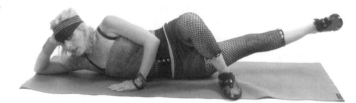

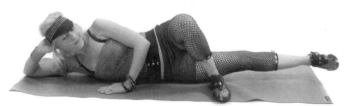

*KEEP THE PRESSURE ON YOUR WORKING INNER THIGH AS YOU RAISE AND LOWER YOUR LEG.

IF PERFORMED WITH ENOUGH DILIGENCE, this exercise will stop your cords from squeaking when you walk.

SCISSOR THIGHS

LEVEL: ☠ ☠

INNER THIGHS

* DON'T LET YOUR LEGS FLOP OPEN.

SLOWLY OPEN THE LEGS AND SLOWLY BRING THEM BACK TOGETHER.

FLEXING THE INNER THIGH MUSCLE.

Lie flat on your back.

Your hands are resting by your sides, palms down.

Extend your legs straight up and point your toes at the ceiling.

Slowly, to a count of eight, spread your legs out to the sides at 45-degree angles to the floor.

At the count of eight, stop your legs from opening any further.

Hold it and flex the foot, and immediately begin counting to eight as you return your legs to the center.

Once they're in their original position, point the toes and begin again.

Do twenty.

Are WE GONNA hAVE TO tEAR you ApArt TO Do tHiS moVe?

THIS ONE will keep your legs looking sharp. We thought we heard J humming a song to this one: "Cause legs...legs will tear us apart...again."

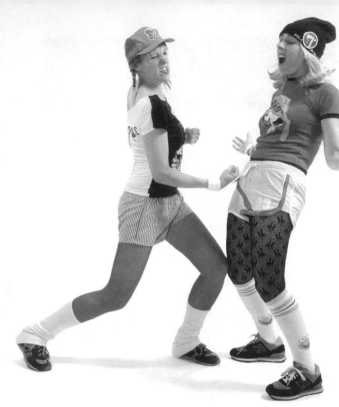

SiX pAcK AnyOnE?

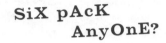

ABs

IF YOU FANTASIZE about having Iggy's washboard abs, but your beer gut gets between you and the ladies, you need to stop munchin' and start crunchin'. We do 120 crunches (combined with other ab exercises) in our class. You have to work up to that, but here are six sets of twenty for you to try, in any order. We suggest that you start with a combination of 60 and add on more as you get stronger. With Iggy as inspiration, you may even lose count and do an extra twenty by mistake!

BuNchEs Of cRUnchEs!

- Push yourself. When you get fatigued and want to stop, try to do three more than you think you can.

- Keep your stomach muscles sucked in while doing these exercises.

- Don't get too worked up over proper breathing techniques. In the beginning, you need to make sure that you don't hold your breath. As you begin to master the exercises, try to incorporate proper breathing technique: exhale on exertion (as you crunch), and inhale as you release (as you roll back to the floor).

- Don't forget to stretch. Always follow your ab work with the Ab Flab stretch from page 2I. It feels great and will keep you from getting sore later on.

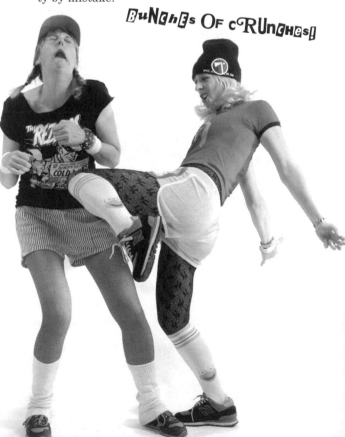

SID-UPS

LEVEL: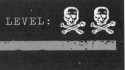

RECTUS ABDOMINIS UPPER (Stomach)

→ KEEP YOUR EYES FOCUSED ON THE CEILING. YOUR WHOLE TORSO SHOULDN'T COME OFF THE FLOOR HERE— IT'S NOT A FULL SIT-UP.

Lie on your back, knees bent and feet flat on the floor, hip-width apart.

Place your hands behind your head to support your neck.

Roll your upper back up off the floor until your shoulders are completely off the floor.

✗ USE YOUR HANDS TO SUPPORT YOUR NECK, NOT TO LIFT YOURSELF HIGHER.

Roll back down, without letting up on the tightness of your upper abs.

As you roll back, your head should barely touch the floor.

Do twenty.

→ FOCUS ON YOUR ABS, KEEPING THEM TIGHT, FEELING THEM WORKING.

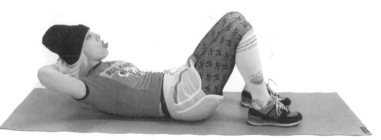

IT'S NOT A REAL, FULL SIT-UP—just a "SID-UP," in homage to Sid Vicious. Anything more formidable would be an insult to his memory...

SUGGESTED LISTENING: "On the Street" by Iggy Pop.

MEET YR KNEE

LEVEL: ☠☠

OBLIQUES (Love Handles)

Ohmigod! i'm lying on the Floor!

Lie on your back, knees bent, feet flat on floor, hip-width apart.

Place one hand behind your head to support your neck.

Your opposite arm is extended to the side supporting you.

i'M gonna touch my Knee!

Roll your upper back off the floor, turning your torso in the direction of the opposite knee—that is, if your left hand is supporting your neck, you want to turn and lift yourself toward your right knee.

Reach toward your knee with your elbow, until your knee and elbow touch.

Slowly roll back down and extend the bent leg straight out.

Do ten sets on each side, for a total of twenty.

...And i Looked Fabulous Doing it!

CENTER CUT

LEVEL: ☠ ☠ ☠

Lie on your back, knees pointed at the ceiling, calves parallel to the floor, with your ankles crossed.

Place your hands behind your head, supporting your neck.

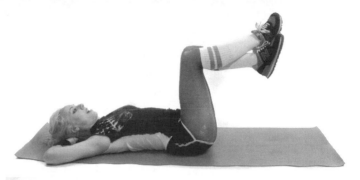

Roll up as if you were doing a simple crunch.

Hold the position for a half second (longer, if you're super-strong).

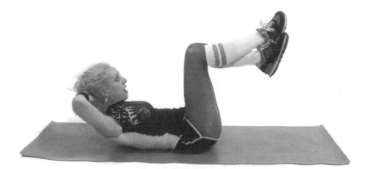

Turn and twist your torso as if you were going to touch the tip of your elbow to the opposite knee.

Return to the center position, staying lifted in a crunch. Slowly lower yourself back down.

Repeat this exercise, turning your torso in the other direction.

Alternate sides with each rep.

Do twenty (ten on each side).

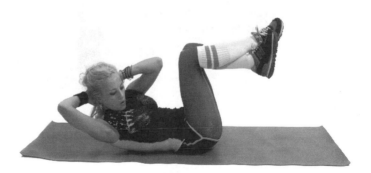

* IT HELPS TO THINK "CENTER, SIDE, CENTER DOWN" AS YOU DO EACH REP. ROLL UP ON CENTER, TURN RIGHT ON SIDE, RETURN TO CENTER ON CENTER, ROLL DOWN ON DOWN. THAT'S ONE REP.

GUT BUSTER

RECTUS ABDOMINIS LOWER (Beer Gut)

Lie with your arms along the side of your body, palms facing down.

Hold your legs up with your knees bent at a 90-degree angle.

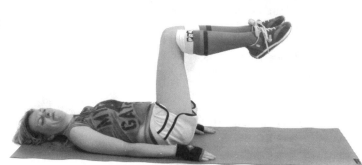

Slowly straighten and lower one of your legs, so that it almost touches the floor.

Hold for half a second and return to your original position: knee bent and your leg at a 90-degree angle.

Repeat with the opposite leg.

Do twenty alternating legs right, left, right, left, and so on.

☆ PRESS THE SMALL OF YOUR BACK TO THE FLOOR AND KEEP YOUR MIND FOCUSED ON YOUR LOWER ABS.

MAURA is wincing in pain because someone stuck a tack under her mat...not 'cause this move hurts. Yeah.

UPSIDE DOWN CROSS

LEVEL: ☠☠

RECTUS ABDOMINIS LOWER (Yr Pot Belly)

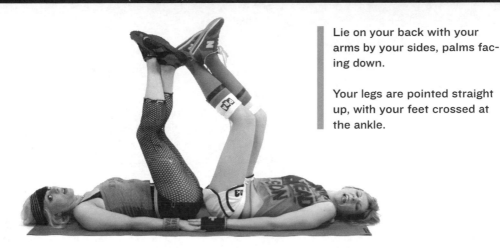

Lie on your back with your arms by your sides, palms facing down.

Your legs are pointed straight up, with your feet crossed at the ankle.

Using your stomach muscles, lift your pelvis and lower back a little bit off the floor.

Lower yourself back down and repeat.

This should be a small, pulsing movement.

Do twenty.

→ DO NOT ✝ USE YOUR ARMS TO SUPPORT YOUR BODY WEIGHT AS YOU LIFT UP, YOU CHEATER!

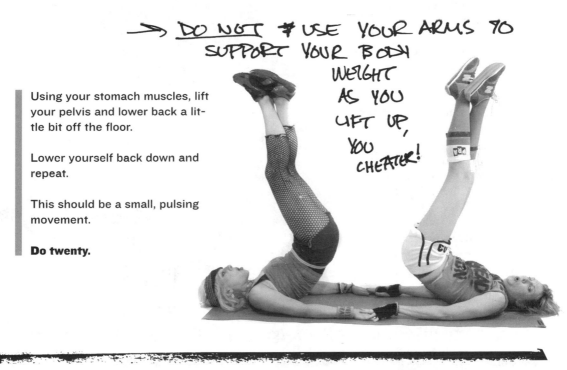

WE THOUGHT WE'D demonstrate this like a punk rock synchronized swimming number.

BICYCLES

RECTUS ABDOMINIS UPPER AND LOWER (The Jelly Roll, Upstairs and Downstairs)

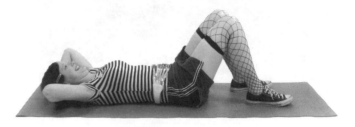

Lie on your back, both hands behind your head and supporting your neck.

Feet are off the floor, knees pointed at the ceiling, calves parallel to the floor.

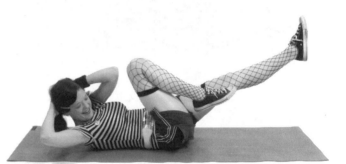

Raise your upper back a few inches off the floor, turning your torso in the direction of the opposite knee.

Reach toward your knee with your elbow.

As you do this, bring your knee in closer to your chest to touch your elbow.

* STAY FOCUSED, AND DO THESE AT A MODERATE PACE...

Roll back down and extend your leg straight out, holding it a few inches above the floor.

Repeat, switching sides right, left, and so on, as if riding a bicycle.

Do twenty.

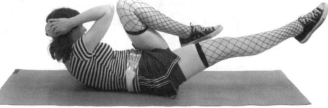

... IT'S EASY TO WANT TO RIP THROUGH THESE, ESPECIALLY IF YOU'RE ROCKING THE TUNES.

MARY TIMONY looks like a pro here—we know she's thinking about whizzing around Boston on a beat up Schwinn.

WATER BOTTLE TORTURE

LEVEL: 💀 💀 💀

RECTUS ABDOMINIS (Lower Abs)

Lie on the floor with your arms propping you up and supporting you.

Your shoulders should be in line with your elbows. Your hands should cup and support your lower back.

With your legs straight out in front of you, put a water bottle (or weight) in-between your feet. Hold it there by squeezing your feet together.

Using your lower abdominals, raise your feet slightly off the ground, and hold the position for a count of ten.

With your hands supporting and holding your lower back, slowly bring your legs back to the starting position.

Do ten.

Repeat.

* KEEP THE PRESSURE ON THOSE LOWER ABS— NOT YOUR BACK, NECK, OR SHOULDERS.

→ YOU MAY WANT TO TAKE A BREAK BETWEEN SETS.

THIS IS ONE OF THOSE MacGyver moments when you can pick up any household item—a water bottle for example—and use it as a weight or a strengthening tool. The goal is to eventually use a 3–5 pound weight.

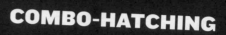

COMBO-HATCHING

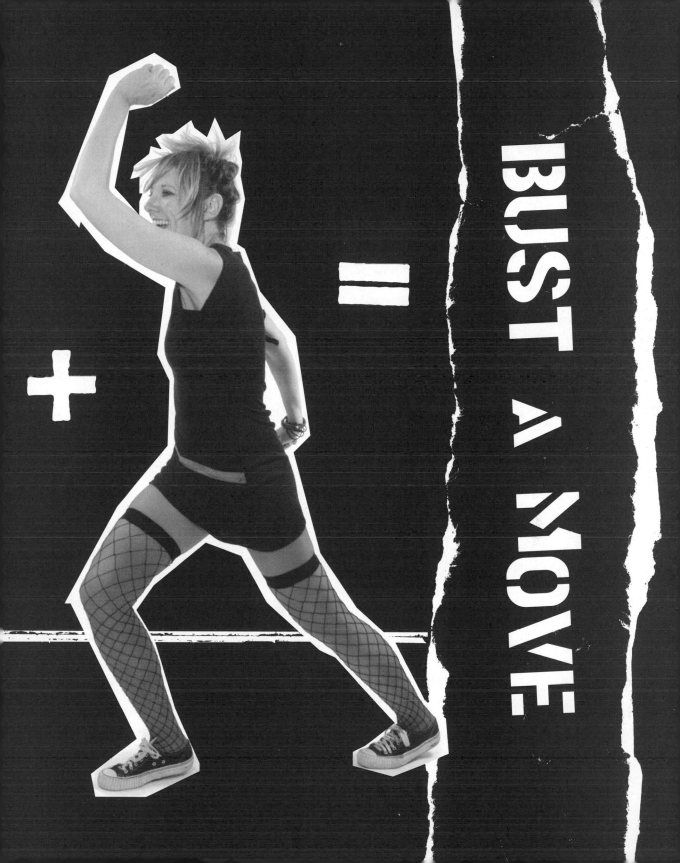

+ = BUST A MOVE

BY NOW, your head might be spinning with the multitude of wild, neck-breaking moves you're about to attempt. It's hard enough to figure out which ones you're capable of executing in your bedroom, never mind before your hysterical roommates, children, or parents as they wander into the living room and point like you're a dancing seal. So you may not be the next Bob Fosse, but there's no need to worry or care. We're going to help you out. Now that we've shown you the moves, it's time to start putting them together, PRA style. You're going to pick some moves and songs to set them to, then you'll be ready to lose yourself in the exquisite mixture of fitness and rock. Here's how we do it…

THE 3 MOVES

JUST LIKE THREE CHORDS in a classic punk song, we pick three moves and set them to a song—otherwise known as *combo-hatching*. For each song, you pick three PRA moves. Now is the time to put that Hi-Fi and Lo-Fi stuff to work. Here's how you do it.

1. Choose two moves that are either Hi-Fi or Lo-Fi—for example, Hi-Fi: Pogo and Rock; Lo-Fi: Side Swipe and Iggy's Punch.

2. If you chose two Hi-Fi moves, choose one Lo-Fi move; if you chose two Lo-Fi moves, choose one move that is Hi-Fi.

Don't pick three Hi-Fi or three Lo-Fi moves—it just doesn't work as well that way. You could have a heart attack if you picked all Hi-Fi moves, or a really low-intensity workout that would do nothing for you if you picked all Lo-Fi moves. (Yes—we are hypocrites with all that talk about doing what you want to do—just obey.)

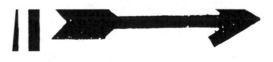

CHOOSE A TUNE

LET'S WALK THROUGH an example of how to pick the three moves and then combo-hatch them.

Flip through the book and find three moves you like a lot, or maybe some that look fun to try. Say you choose **You Be the Star Air Guitar** ('cause you're revving up for your big Jimmy Page tribute at the local karaoke bar), **Iggy's Pop** (because he's your favorite and you like the name), and the **Hip Slug** (because your dad just had a hip replacement and that's what you've been calling him behind his back). There you go—you've picked two Hi-Fi moves and one Lo-Fi move. Great combo-hatch!

You're almost there, now you've got to put them to music!

NOW THAT YOU'VE GOT YOUR MOVES, it's time to pick the tune that you want to set them to. Start out by picking a really great song—I mean, that's how Punk Rock Aerobics got started in the first place. When we pushed that coffee table over and started pogoing like crazy, it wasn't because Art Garfunkel was shaking the floorboards. You need to pick a song that makes you lose control. One that you know from experience is going to work some Jekyll and Hyde magic and turn you into a monster of rock. As we mentioned in the beginning, you'll want to have twenty to forty minutes of songs on a tape or CD; but for now, pick one great song you'd take to a desert island and blast it!

IT LOOKS LIKE THIS:

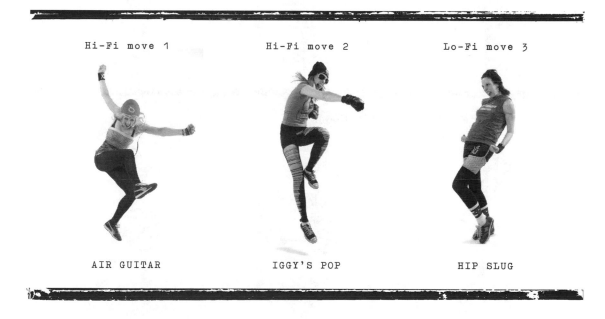

Hi-Fi move 1   Hi-Fi move 2   Lo-Fi move 3

AIR GUITAR   IGGY'S POP   HIP SLUG

COMBO-HATCHING ACTION

NOW THAT YOU'VE GOT the three moves and you've picked a tune, it's time to give combo-hatching a try. Putting the moves to song might feel awkward at first, but remember—there's no right or wrong way to do it; all moves are not going to go with all songs. Make sure that the moves you've chosen feel good with the tempo of the tune you've picked. For example, if you picked "Pay to Cum" by the Bad Brains, it's obviously going to be hard to do much of anything besides Skank. Use your brain—it's a muscle too. You may need to experiment a little and figure out if that Sideswipe fits with your favorite Buzzcocks song. Or maybe play one of your favorite CDs and go through some of our moves to find out which ones fit best.

OUR FAVORITE COMBO-HATCHES

HERE ARE SOME EXAMPLES OF SONGS AND MOVES TO SET TO THEM.

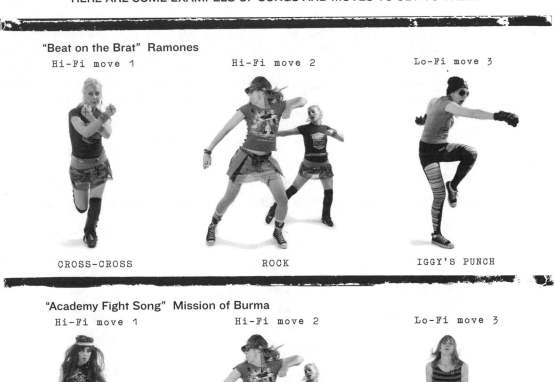

"Beat on the Brat" Ramones

Hi-Fi move 1 — CROSS-CROSS

Hi-Fi move 2 — ROCK

Lo-Fi move 3 — IGGY'S PUNCH

"Academy Fight Song" Mission of Burma

Hi-Fi move 1 — SWIZZLE SWISH

Hi-Fi move 2 — ROCK

Lo-Fi move 3 — SIDESWIPE

"Seventeen Years of Hell" Partisans

Lo-Fi move 1   Lo-Fi move 2   Hi-Fi move 3

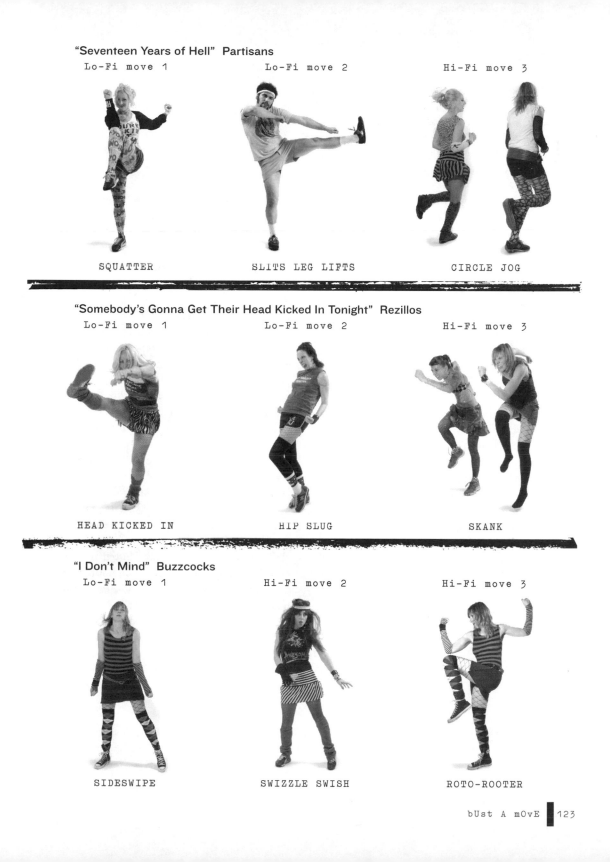

SQUATTER   SLITS LEG LIFTS   CIRCLE JOG

"Somebody's Gonna Get Their Head Kicked In Tonight" Rezillos

Lo-Fi move 1   Lo-Fi move 2   Hi-Fi move 3

HEAD KICKED IN   HIP SLUG   SKANK

"I Don't Mind" Buzzcocks

Lo-Fi move 1   Hi-Fi move 2   Hi-Fi move 3

SIDESWIPE   SWIZZLE SWISH   ROTO-ROOTER

AS WE MENTIONED EARLIER, you may be asking yourself, "Why don't I just jump up and down to any old song? Why the whole three moves thing? Who cares?" Well, the three moves will help give a little more structure to your routine, so that you get the kind of workout that is right for you, and that actually works a lot better than random jumping up and down. You can use the three moves to make songs easier or harder, gradually building in intensity as you go, then lowering the intensity as you begin cooling down at the end of your workout. You can pick moves that work a muscle group more specifically, and will strengthen muscles as you go (for example, Bacne, Slits Leg Lift, Thin Thighs). These cardio moves are more than just about pogoing—they work to strengthen body parts a little bit more than the usual freak-scene dance party, and add more power (and sometimes difficulty) to your workout.

If jumping around is all that you're up for, though, that's cool with us. Go nuts with some basic cardio moves such as Pogo, Skank, and Wack Jack. If you want to do a bunch of Hi-Fi moves together and just not deal with putting in more effort, have fun and knock yourself out. You'll get your heart rate up, you'll be exercising, and that's all we care about. Or stay there sitting on the couch and have a dance party in your pants. Hey, whatever works.

TWENTY-MINUTE ROCK BLOCKS!

HERE'S WHERE IT GETS COOL—and a little bit hard too. No more kiddie school, with one song at a time. We're putting the songs together now. No stopping in between 'em and let's go.

The point here is to do a cardio workout that lasts for twenty minutes. So if you have six songs in your twenty-minute rock block and each song has three moves, then you are doing eighteen moves in total. That's a whole lot of movin' and groovin' and shakin'. But I guess that's the whole point.

Now all you need to do is to find some of your favorite songs. Whip out that calculator and make sure that they add up to twenty minutes. That's all the time you need to get your cardio done—you don't need to be a brain surgeon when it comes to this one.

We have provided a list of perfectly formed punk rock blocks, where all you have to do is pick your three moves for each song and stick them in. Just to show you, we'll give you an example of three moves you can combo-hatch in each song, and that way, you can try it and not have to come up with them all by your lonesome. Unless you feel like you're ready, go ahead and pick 'em yourself. After that, we'll show you the song list with the running times next to it, so you can see for yourself that you have done your PRA cardio combo-hatching for a full twenty minutes. Then you can be proud of yourself afterward.

A TWENTY MINUTE ROCK-BLOCK

EACH COMBO-HATCH HAS A GOOD MIX OF LO-FI AND HI-FI MOVES, SO YOU GET AN EVEN WORKOUT.

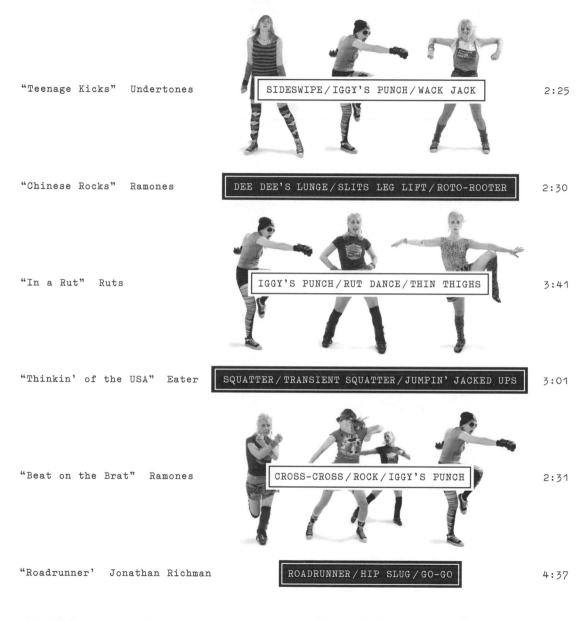

"Teenage Kicks" Undertones — SIDESWIPE / IGGY'S PUNCH / WACK JACK — 2:25

"Chinese Rocks" Ramones — DEE DEE'S LUNGE / SLITS LEG LIFT / ROTO-ROOTER — 2:30

"In a Rut" Ruts — IGGY'S PUNCH / RUT DANCE / THIN THIGHS — 3:41

"Thinkin' of the USA" Eater — SQUATTER / TRANSIENT SQUATTER / JUMPIN' JACKED UPS — 3:01

"Beat on the Brat" Ramones — CROSS-CROSS / ROCK / IGGY'S PUNCH — 2:31

"Roadrunner' Jonathan Richman — ROADRUNNER / HIP SLUG / GO-GO — 4:37

TOTAL RUNNING TIME 18:45

ROCK-BLOCKS ON THE GO

WE KNOW that most of you don't want to sit around timing songs, so we've decided to do some of the work for you by providing a list of some of our favorites tunes, the band that performs them, and the running times. This is a great way to help you to put together your rock block in a hurry.

SONGS TO PICK FOR YOUR PUNK ROCK TWENTY-MINUTE SONG BLOCK, STRENGTH TRAINING, AND STRETCHING.

SONG	BAND	TIME
"Mannequin"	Wire	2:37
"Shot from Both Sides"	Magazine	4:01
"L.A."	The Fall	4:09
"Look, Know"	The Fall	4:48
"No Fun"	The Stooges	5:15
"TV Eye"	The Stooges	4:17
"Search and Destroy"	The Stooges	3:26
"Public Image"	PIL	6:05
"What Do I Get?"	Buzzcocks	2:52
"Why Can't I Touch It?"	Buzzcocks	6:32
"Everybody's Happy Nowadays"	Buzzcocks	3:09
"Ever Fallen in Love"	Buzzcocks	2:39
"Promises"	Buzzcocks	2:34
"Lipstick"	Buzzcocks	2:36
"God Save the Queen"	Sex Pistols	3:18
"Better Off Dead"	Wipers	5:10
"ha ha ha"	Flipper	4:03
"Little Babies"	Sleater Kinney	2:19
"Teenage Kicks"	Undertones	2:25
"Blitzkrieg Bop"	Ramones	2:14
"Chinese Rocks"	Ramones	2:30
"Beat on the Brat"	Ramones	2:31
"Do the Boob"	The Real Kids	2:16
"You've Got My Number"	Undertones	3:00
"In a Rut"	Ruts	3:41
"Seventeen Years of Hell"	Partisans	2:50
"Gary Gilmore's Eyes"	Adverts	2:11
"Sonic Reducer"	Dead Boys	3:05
"Freak Scene"	Dinosaur Jr.	3:35
"Thinkin' of the USA"	Eater	3:01
"Hate Breeders"	Misfits	3:00
"All Hell Breaks Loose"	Misfits	1:47
"I Turned into a Martian"	Misfits	1:43
"Somebody's Gonna Get Their Head Kicked In Tonight"	Rezillos	2:11
"Unite and Fight as One"	FU's	2:00
"Roadrunner"	Jonathan Richman	4:37
"Love Song"	Damned	2:00
"That's How I Escaped My Certain Fate"	Mission of Burma	2:03
"Trem Two"	Mission of Burma	4:10
"Pay to Cum"	Bad Brains	1:25
"The Big Takeover"	Bad Brains	2:57

VINYL WORKOUTS

If you want to start scouring your local record stores for rarities that feature the best in vintage aerobic activity, here are some personal favorites.

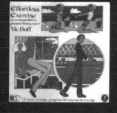

EFFORTLESS EXERCISE,
AS RECOMMENDED BY PHYSICAL FITNESS EXPERT VIC BOFF
This work refers to itself as a total exercise program for anyone at any age. The workouts are designed for a person who has no time and, clearly, no energy. Vic likes to tell you the ways in which you can get a stretch while doing the dishes or getting up from a chair. It also comes with a great book full of seventies-era cartoon illustrations. Boff sounds as though he downed a bottle of valium before he went in to the studio. Rock!

JENNY SCANDIFF'S AEROBIC LIFESTYLE
Anyone who says, "Come on, smile—burn those bottoms" ought to have her bottom burned with a branding iron. Accompanied by a booklet that includes recipes such as "Super Fruit Soup." It looks like Super Fruit Poop. No thanks, I'll have a smoothie.

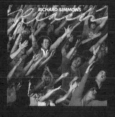

REACH, BY RICHARD SIMMONS
You can laugh all you want, but Simmons is a creative genius. This record is better and more fun to listen to than most of the crap out there. The songs sound like something you'd hear on Sesame Street backed with disco-era synthesizers and percussion. It comes with a booklet full of cool photos and a warning that reads, "The shrink wrap on this album has been treated with an invisible substance that measures perspiration. If you're not sweating enough, an electronic laser will zap out of your stereo system and pinch your tushy." Bust out your leotard and crack open a beer.

JOHN DEVLIN'S STRETCH OUT EXERCISE CLASS
This album sounds uncannily like a song called "The Gift" by the Velvet Underground, which tells the story of a sad sack named Waldo who crawls into a box and mails himself to his girlfriend, who lives in a different state. When the box arrives, she has trouble getting it open, reaches for a knife, and unwittingly stabs poor Waldo to death. Devlin's record features music and narration so similar to those on "The Gift" that we suspect Lou Reed was doing his daily workout to it when he wrote that song. Listen to it on painkillers and it will freak you out.

6

CREATING
THE PERFECT WORKOUT

SLAPPIN' IT

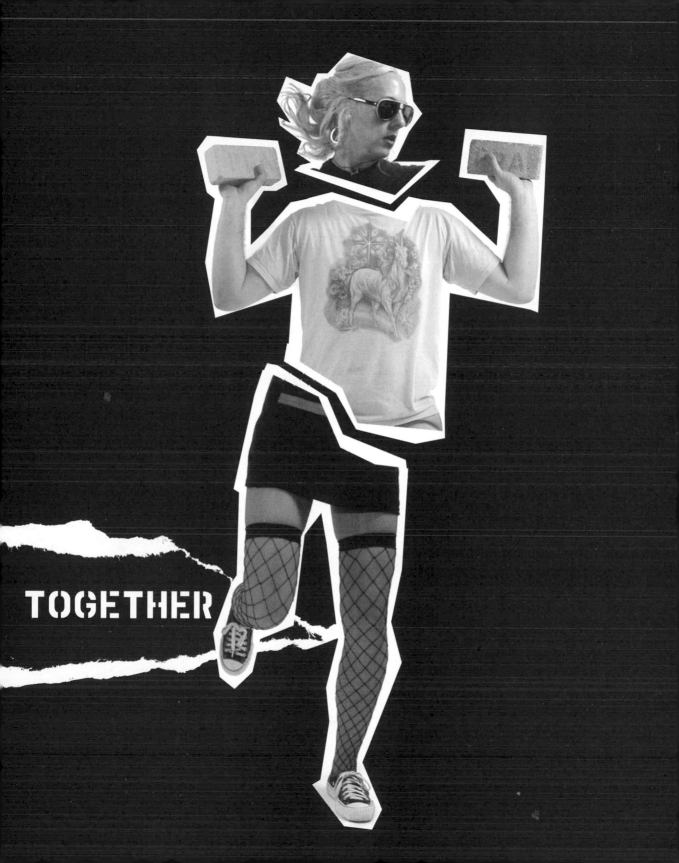

TOGETHER

STRETCHING, CARDIO, AND STRENGTH TRAINING. By now, you're probably wondering how the three elements work together. When do you put the stretching in? How long should you strength train, or use the weights, and how many exercises should you do? How long does cardio really need to be? We're going to review the key elements of the workout and show you some sample workouts of different time lengths, for all you busy workaholics or sods on the dole.

STRETCHING

BEGIN YOUR WORKOUT with some basic stretches for your upper and lower body. Keep them simple. We recommend picking an equal number of stretches from each. For example: Moron Rollup / Gas Bag / Ham Sandwich Stretch / Mono Leg / Cat Scratch Fever / Leaning Tower of Torso / Neck-Breaka. Cover all your bases. At the end of your workout, when your body is warmed up, your muscles will be more responsive to stretches. Stretching is also a great way to release tension and slowly return to a more chill state of mind after all that angst-fueled skanking. If you have time, we recommend five to ten minutes of stretching to start, and ten or more minutes of stretching at the end of your workout. Keep in mind, stretching can be done every day.

Got it? Start with five minutes at the beginning of your workout, and ten minutes at the end. You can stretch every day.

CARDIO

THE CARDIO PART of the workout should be heavy on fun. At this point, you only need to decide how long you want to spend on cardio, and how hard you want it to be. We recommend a twenty-minute minimum rock block to start, but no one is going to care if you can only handle ten minutes in the beginning. Just do what you can, and work up to the optimum amount. Unless you're interested in building endurance, it doesn't matter if you do forty minutes at once or twenty minutes twice—we prefer intensity over endurance. Yet you may want to build endurance so that you've got all the stamina you'll need the next time you outrun security after you steal a fitness book from Tower Records.

HOWEVER LONG YOUR WORKOUT, you'll want to control the level of intensity, working from a moderate pace to a fast pace, then slowing the pace as you cool down. How will you do this? By using lots of Lo-Fi moves at the beginning of your workout and incorporating the harder, more intense Hi-Fi moves in the middle and throughout. As you start to bring your cardio workout to an end, use songs with more Lo-Fi moves, making the last song as simple and low key as you can (within limits—there's no need for a key as low as Phil Collins). It's important to do this so that you can bring your heart rate down gradually. Unless you don't mind passing out during the daytime or dropping dead from heart failure, we don't recommend that you eliminate a proper cool-down period from your workout. Got it?

Do twenty minutes of cardio if you can. If you want to add on to that, go ahead. Make sure that your first couple of songs start slow (Lo-Fi) and build in intensity (Hi-Fi). When you are ready to wind down, make sure that you have at least one song with slower (Lo-Fi) moves at the end. You can do a cardio workout every day.

STRENGTH TRAINING

STRENGTH TRAINING CAN BE DONE alone or as part of your overall workout, but you'll get the best results by doing it after you've warmed up with some aerobic activity. Spending ten to twenty minutes on strength training three to four times a week will do the trick, to start. Don't strength train every day; you need to rest a day or two in between for your muscles to rebuild, or they'll be damaged goods. Just 'cause Gang of Four says "send them back" doesn't mean you'll be able to. So give it a break and go pick some flowers or do your hair or something....

Do at least ten to twenty minutes of strength training three to four times a week. Don't strength train daily.

Even though we want you to be able to create your very own workout, here are some samples to help you get started. Let's begin with the workout as we do it in our class. Of course, you won't get the pleasure of watching us mess it up or make fun of one another, but we trust that you'll find your own clever ways to keep it fun.

THE P.R.A. CORPORATE PROCEDURE WORKOUT

THIS IS THE FULL, ONE-HOUR PRA workout (not including stretching time) from our class. We begin with stretching, move on to cardio once you're warmed up, break it up with strength, sock you with more cardio, bring you back to strength, and cool you down. Phew!

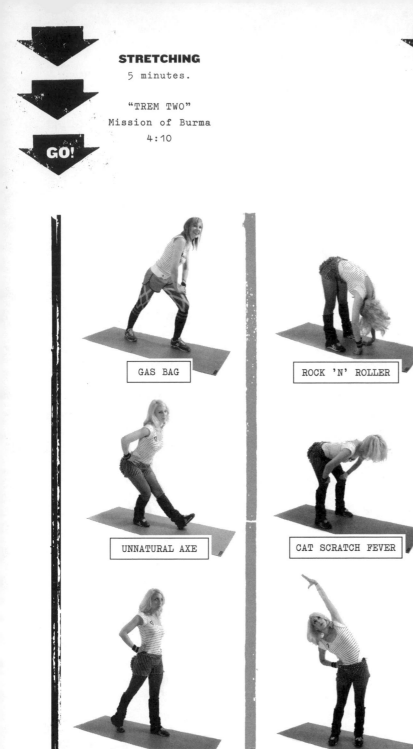

STRETCHING

5 minutes.

"TREM TWO"
Mission of Burma
4:10

GO!

GAS BAG

ROCK 'N' ROLLER

UNNATURAL AXE

CAT SCRATCH FEVER

MORON ROLLUP

LEANING TOWER OF TORSO

CARDIO

20 minutes.

Begin with two songs most
suitable for Lo-Fi.
Here are a few examples:

"TEENAGE KICKS"
Undertones 2:25

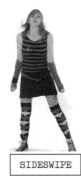

SIDESWIPE

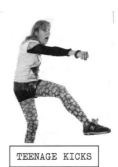

TEENAGE KICKS

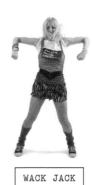

WACK JACK

Continue with songs
suitable for Hi-Fi.
The following, for example:

"CHINESE ROCKS"　　　　　"IN A RUT"　　　　　"I DON'T MIND"
Heartbreakers 2:30　　　　Ruts 3:41　　　　Buzzcocks 2:20

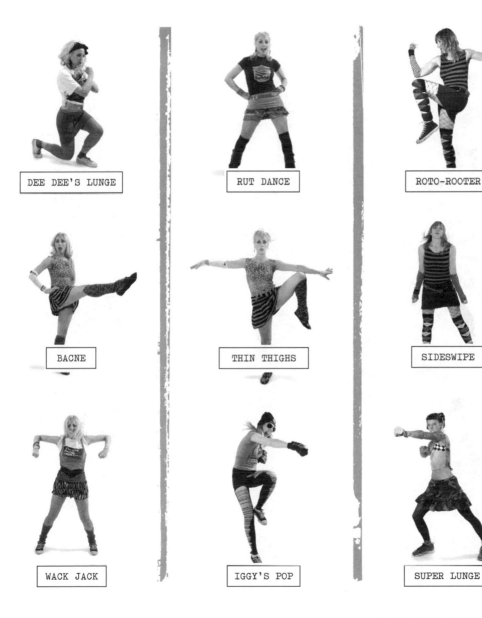

DEE DEE'S LUNGE　　　RUT DANCE　　　ROTO-ROOTER

BACNE　　　THIN THIGHS　　　SIDESWIPE

WACK JACK　　　IGGY'S POP　　　SUPER LUNGE

Continue with one or
two songs suitable
for Lo-Fi. For example,
the following:

"BEAT ON THE BRAT"
Ramones 2:31

"ROADRUNNER"
Jonathan Richman 4:37

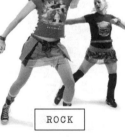

CROSS-CROSS

ROADRUNNER

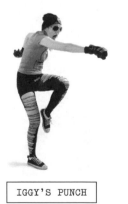

ROCK

GO-GO

IGGY'S PUNCH

POGO

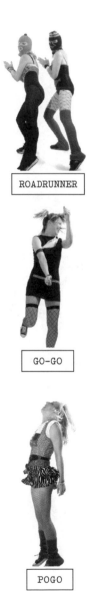

* REMEMBER, IT WORKS BETTER IF YOU DON'T DO ALL LOFI MOVES OR ALL HI-FI MOVES TO ANY SONG. WHEN WE SAY A SONG IS GOOD FOR LO-FI WE MEAN IT'S GOOD FOR A COMBINATION OF 2 LO-FI MOVES AND 1 HI-FI MOVE. WHEN WE SAY A SONG IS GOOD FOR HI-FI, WE MEAN IT'S GOOD FOR A COMBINATION OF 2 HI-FI MOVES AND 1 LO-FI.

STRENGTH TRAINING
Set I
5 minutes.

CARDIO
20 minutes.

**Begin with one song
suitable for Lo-Fi.**

"GOD SAVE THE QUEEN"
Sex Pistols 3:18

**Continue with songs
suitable for Hi-Fi:**

"LITTLE BABIES"
Sleater-Kinney 2:13

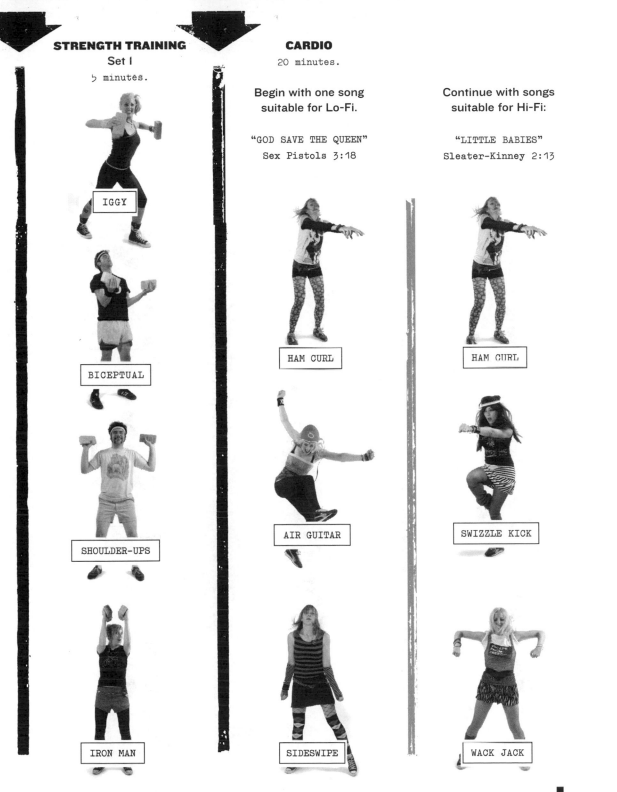

IGGY

BICEPTUAL

SHOULDER-UPS

IRON MAN

HAM CURL

AIR GUITAR

SIDESWIPE

HAM CURL

SWIZZLE KICK

WACK JACK

"FREAK SCENE"
Dinosaur Jr. 3:35

"SOMEBODY'S GONNA GET
THEIR HEAD
KICKED IN TONIGHT"
Rezillos 1:53

"TYPICAL GIRLS"
Slits 3:50

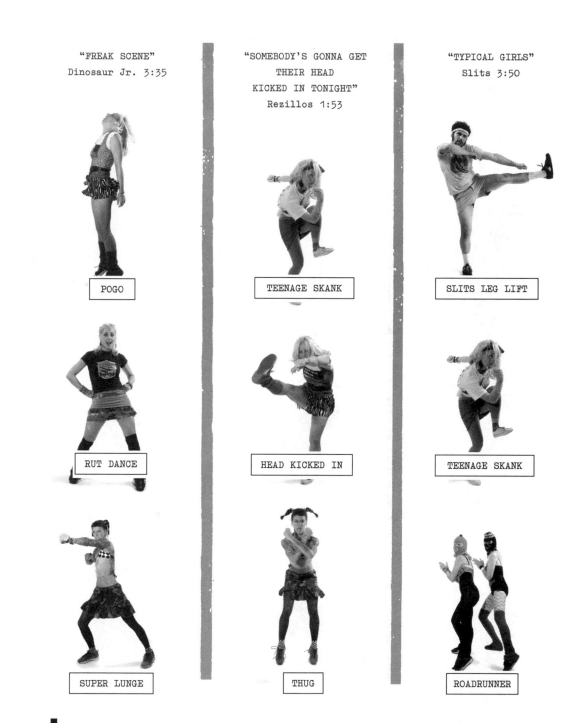

POGO

TEENAGE SKANK

SLITS LEG LIFT

RUT DANCE

HEAD KICKED IN

TEENAGE SKANK

SUPER LUNGE

THUG

ROADRUNNER

STRENGTH TRAINING
Set 2
15 minutes.

Now for fifteen minutes
of weights and mat work
(exercises you do
on the floor with a mat).

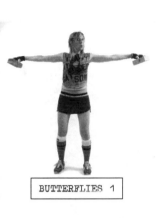

BUTTERFLIES 1

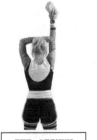

THE STINKY

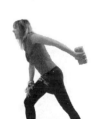

CHICKEN WING 1

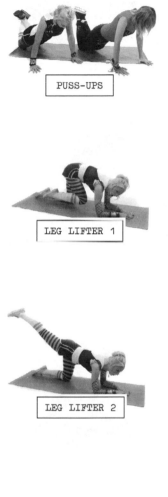

PUSS-UPS

LEG LIFTER 1

LEG LIFTER 2

LEG LIFTER 3

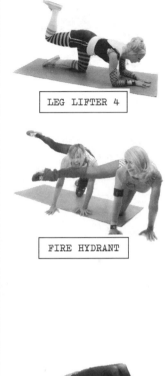

LEG LIFTER 4

FIRE HYDRANT

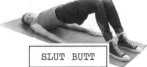

SLUT BUTT

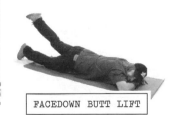

FACEDOWN BUTT LIFT

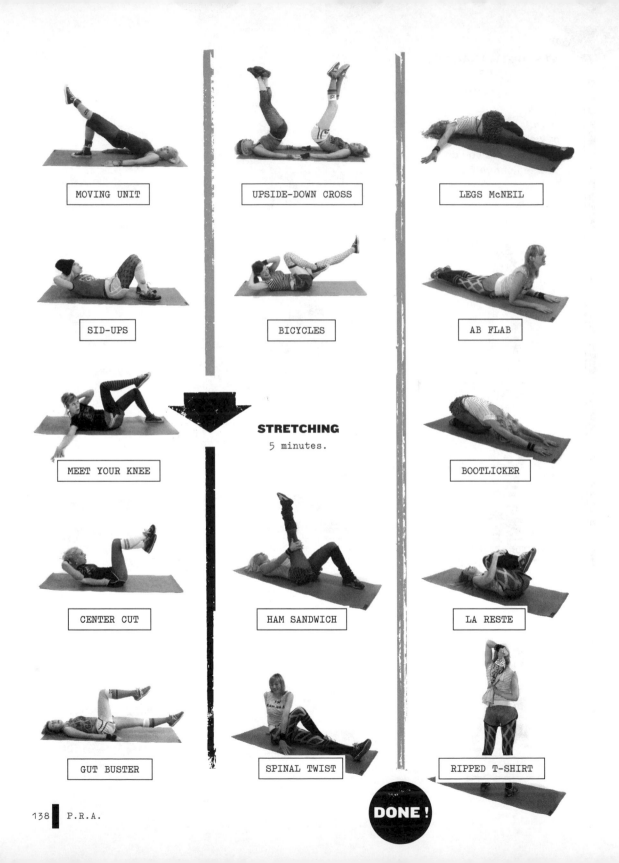

MOVING UNIT

UPSIDE-DOWN CROSS

LEGS McNEIL

SID-UPS

BICYCLES

AB FLAB

STRETCHING

5 minutes.

MEET YOUR KNEE

BOOTLICKER

CENTER CUT

HAM SANDWICH

LA RESTE

GUT BUSTER

SPINAL TWIST

RIPPED T-SHIRT

DONE !

OUT OF TIME

SHORTER WORKOUTS FOR THE HARRIED

SO WE'VE JUST SHOWN YOU the standard PRA blueprint, the one-hour workout we do in our classes. Let's take a moment to answer two predictable objections.

OBJECTION #1:

YOU: Who besides Madonna would want to spend an hour a day on her body?

US: In our class, we feel that an hour goes by quickly—if all goes well, it turns into a dance party. The reason why we pay such close attention to the music is that we want to make you lose track of time. You can't listen to the ticking of the clock when you're listening to Gang of Four rip through "Damaged Goods" during a weight-lifting section. "Sweat's running down your neck/Sweat's running down your back." When you hear that stuff, it's just too good to pay attention or to care about anything else at that point, especially the pain the Biceptual is causing you.

OBJECTION #2:

YOU: Only Madonna HAS an hour a day to work on her body.

US: Fine, we can't help you here. We don't expect you to behave like you're the chairman of MGM and work out from six to seven in the morning before you lock yourself in the office for fourteen hours. So we've mapped out some shorter workouts.

THE P.R.A. ONE-CARDIO-WAVE WORKOUT

This routine covers your whole body in no more than forty minutes. It's like the hour-long PRA Corporate Procedure Workout, except for the following changes:

- you only do one twenty-minute cardio block;
- you begin and end with only four stretching exercises;
- you have a shorter strength-training session—just pick two of our three strength-training categories (ass, abs, arms), then pick three exercises from each.

GO!

Here's an example of a One-Cardio-Wave Workout.

STRETCHING
5 minutes.

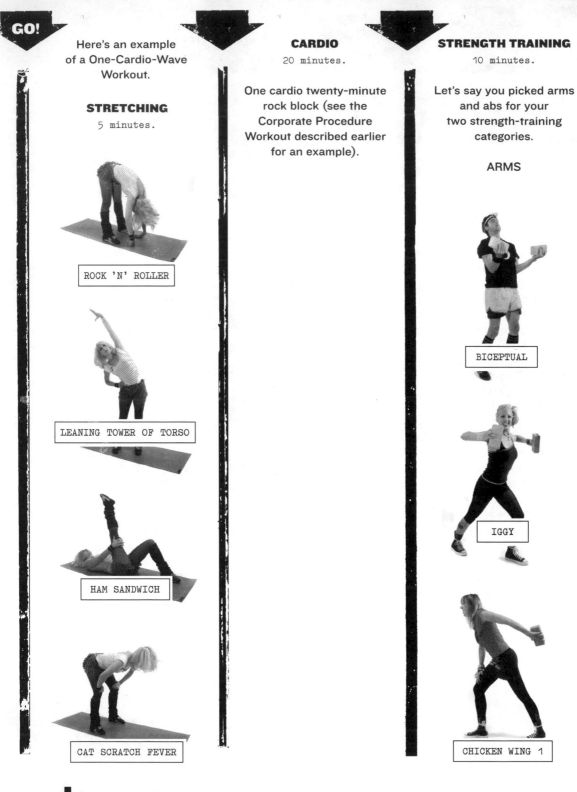

ROCK 'N' ROLLER

LEANING TOWER OF TORSO

HAM SANDWICH

CAT SCRATCH FEVER

CARDIO
20 minutes.

One cardio twenty-minute rock block (see the Corporate Procedure Workout described earlier for an example).

STRENGTH TRAINING
10 minutes.

Let's say you picked arms and abs for your two strength-training categories.

ARMS

BICEPTUAL

IGGY

CHICKEN WING 1

ABS

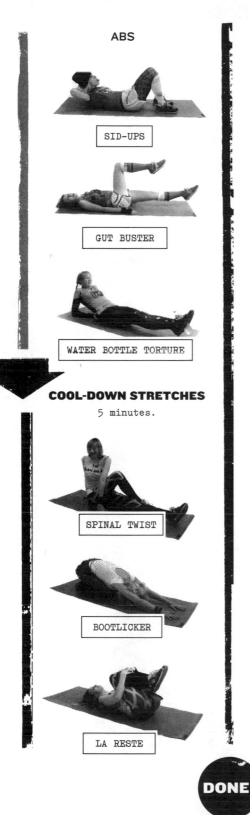

SID-UPS

GUT BUSTER

WATER BOTTLE TORTURE

COOL-DOWN STRETCHES
5 minutes.

SPINAL TWIST

BOOTLICKER

LA RESTE

DONE !

THE P.R.A. HALF-HOUR WORKOUT

"FORTY MINUTES?" you gasp. "My grandmother doesn't have forty min—Christ, I have to take this call." Never fear. We've heard that a mere thirty minutes of exercise a day is one of the easiest ways to ensure better health for the future. It's a short amount of time for a serious return in life expectancy. So we say do it. If you don't have time for even half an hour, well, who knows what the health mags will say next? Screw 'em. Flip through the pictures in this book while you walk around the block or something.

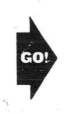

GO!

Here's an example of a half-hour PRA workout.

STRETCHING
2 minutes.

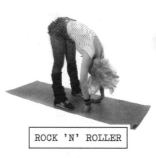

ROCK 'N' ROLLER

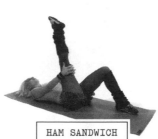

HAM SANDWICH

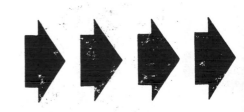

CARDIO
15 minutes.

This has to be heavy on the Hi-Fi the entire time, because it's short and you can probably only play a few tunes. We suggest the following:

"YOU'VE GOT MY NUMBER"
The Undertones 3:00

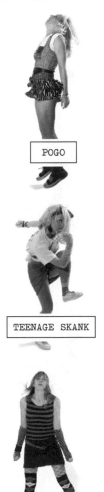

POGO

TEENAGE SKANK

SIDESWIPE

"LOVE SONG"
The Damned 2:00

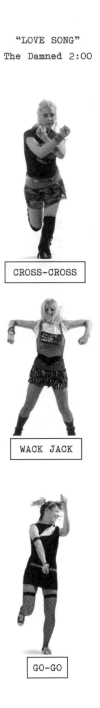

CROSS-CROSS

WACK JACK

GO-GO

"MANNEQUIN"
Wire 2:37

TEENAGE SKANK

PLUNGER

SWIZZLE SWISH

"EVER FALLEN IN LOVE"	"MY OLD MAN'S A FATSO"	"TONGUE TIED"
Buzzcocks 2:39	Angry Samoans 1:29	Erase Erata 1:38

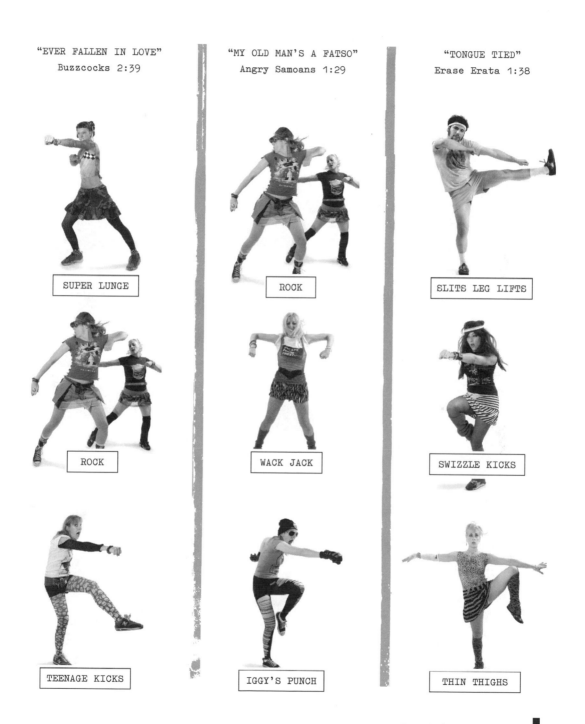

SUPER LUNGE	ROCK	SLITS LEG LIFTS
ROCK	WACK JACK	SWIZZLE KICKS
TEENAGE KICKS	IGGY'S PUNCH	THIN THIGHS

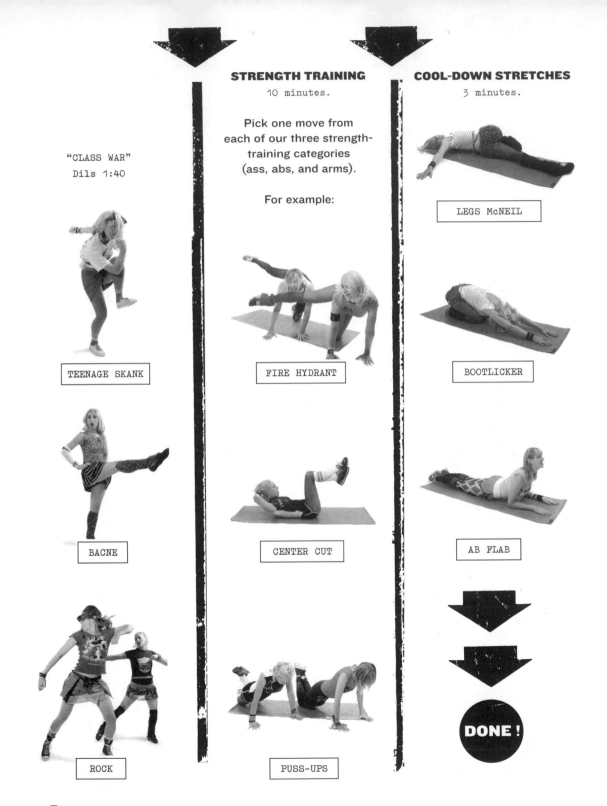

STRENGTH TRAINING

10 minutes.

Pick one move from each of our three strength-training categories (ass, abs, and arms).

For example:

COOL-DOWN STRETCHES

3 minutes.

"CLASS WAR"
Dils 1:40

LEGS McNEIL

TEENAGE SKANK

FIRE HYDRANT

BOOTLICKER

BACNE

CENTER CUT

AB FLAB

ROCK

PUSS-UPS

DONE !

THE P.R.A. STRENGTH-TRAINING ONLY WORKOUT

THIS ROUTINE WORKS ALL THE MUSCLE GROUPS IN YOUR BODY USING WEIGHTS AND MAT EXERCISES, FOR THOSE DAYS WHEN YOU WANT TO BLOW OFF CARDIO.

PICK FOUR EXERCISES FROM EACH STRENGTH-TRAINING CATEGORY.
HERE'S AN EXAMPLE:

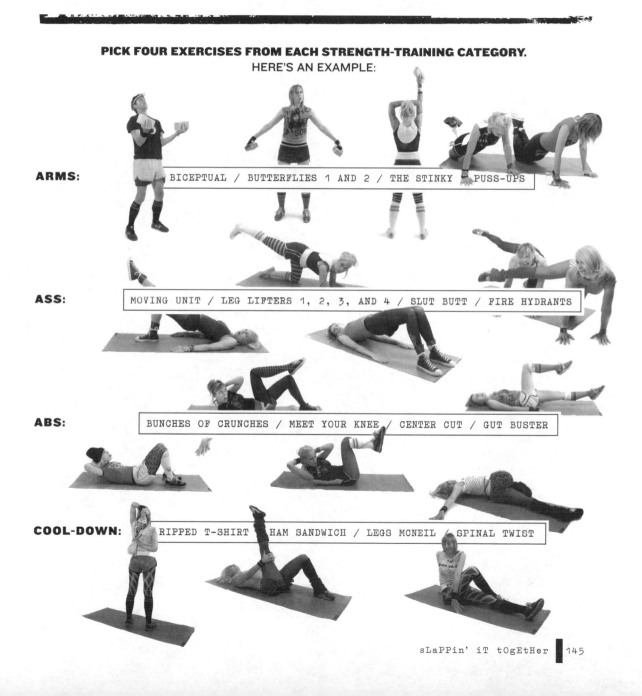

ARMS: BICEPTUAL / BUTTERFLIES 1 AND 2 / THE STINKY / PUSS-UPS

ASS: MOVING UNIT / LEG LIFTERS 1, 2, 3, AND 4 / SLUT BUTT / FIRE HYDRANTS

ABS: BUNCHES OF CRUNCHES / MEET YOUR KNEE / CENTER CUT / GUT BUSTER

COOL-DOWN: RIPPED T-SHIRT / HAM SANDWICH / LEGS MCNEIL / SPINAL TWIST

Robyn Hitchcock

The Soft Boys

....

When you think about getting into shape, does it make you think you have to radically change your lifestyle?

Every time I change my lifestyle, my shape alters, yes, it's true. And to me it's tragic that you can't smoke in New York any more. The Jazz Age is really over. Roll on, Miller Lite and the world of airport sports bars. Hey, maybe Bush'll get in again. Not that he smokes. Oh no. But William Burroughs did.

Do you have a gym membership?

Not currently, but I have had one for several years. Unfortunately, touring disrupts my exercise routines and replaces them with alcohol and tobacco. But you will note that this hasn't happened to Henry Rollins.

Do you think William S. Burroughs ever lifted a weight in his life?

He lifted cats, and cats can weigh up to 120 pounds. Burroughs was an Aquarius, and they're an unfathomable crew.

If you exercise, what type of exercise do you do? And what kind of music do you listen to when working out?

The cycling machine brings you out in a breathless sweat, so that's fun. But I'm drifting towards yoga. Swimming is reliable, but I haven't yet found an underwater walkman. Is there one? As a rule, listening to music from when you were young makes you feel more energetic. I can really break a sweat listening to the Dave Clark Five. "Walking On Sunshine" is good for the heart, too.

Have you ever pushed away the coffee table to dance until all hours of the morning? What songs or records have inspired you to physically move?

As a rule, no. I tend to vibrate internally, like the Flash, so you don't see me move much. I hope eventually to be able to pass through solid objects, for instance Mount Rushmore. Sometimes I dance when Grant-Lee Phillips plays the guitar and we perform Philly Soul classics like "Rock Your Baby."

Does Natalie Merchant's interpretive dancing inspire you?

Only to homicide.

Is Frisbee a sport to you or just a major at Hampshire College?

It's something other people do.

If you're on the road and one of your bandmates or fellow touring bands gets up to go for a jog, do you hate them or join them?

I admire them. Kimberley Rew goes jogging most mornings. He wrote "Walking On Sunshine."

Has your state of "being in shape" ever affected your performance either positively or negatively? Do you tend to work up a sweat onstage?

No, although I tend to sweat out the previous night's alcohol onstage. Or that afternoon's coffee. Thank you for taking an interest in my glands.

Do you like your body, or are you among the ranks of people who think that if they could just lose those ten pounds, they'd be perfect?

Probably losing 14 pounds would help. I am my body, but I haven't fully realized that yet. We tend to think we're driving ourselves, like cars but we are the actual vehicles. Not that this rules out soul-transference or reincarnation.

As a performer in the public eye, has body image ever been a concern? Have you ever had outside pressure (i.e., from a label, etc) about your weight/shape?

No, but the *San Francisco Chronicle* said I looked pregnant when I played there on the Soft Boys tour. I renewed my gym membership that year.

Do you think that fat people get no respect?

Well, there's plenty of them, so that's a shame if it's true. It's harder for women, in all this; men (or at least, hetero men) are under less pressure to be conventionally attractive than women are. According to the latest statistics, 75% of Americans are obese, 24.999999% are anorexic, and the other two are Brad Pitt and Jennifer Aniston, representing the correct physique. Can you imagine the pressure those two are under?

THE P.R.A. CRAZY CARDIO WORKOUT

THIS IS A ROUTINE for those who want to bushwhack through forty minutes of heat-pumping aerobic exercise. Make a set of your favorite tunes that adds up to forty minutes in length (two rock blocks), and then, as per usual, make up a combo-hatch of moves for each song. Keep in mind that you will need to stretch and warm up your body before you jump in. And remember, your last song needs to be a little slower than the rest of the songs so that you can cool off to it.

HERE'S A SAMPLE CRAZY CARDIO ROUTINE:

SONG/BAND	TIME	THREE MOVES TO COMBO-HATCH
"READ ABOUT SEYMOUR," Swell Maps	1:25	AIR GUITAR/PLUNGER/SWIZZLE SWISH
"1977," The Clash	1:40	TRANSIENT SQUATTER/ROADRUNNER/THUG
"PROSTITUTES," The Pop Group	3:10	SIDESWIPE/THIN THIGHS/WACK JACKS
"TV EYE," The Stooges	4:17	ROTO-ROOTER/POGO/BACNE
"ONE CHORD WONDERS," The Adverts	2:43	CROSS-CROSS/IGGY'S PUNCH/TEENAGE KICK
"DIG ME OUT," Sleater-Kinney	2:37	TRANSIENT SQUATTER/SWIZZLE KICKS/AIR GUITAR
"AMBITION," Vic Godard	2:58	SLITS LEG LIFTS/GO-GO/JUMPIN' JACKED UPS
"PSYCHO MAFIA," The Fall	2:12	POGO/ROTO-ROOTER/IGGY'S PUNCH
"EVER FALLEN IN LOVE," Buzzcocks	2:39	CROSS-CROSS/ROCK/TEENAGE KICK
"EX-LION TAMER," Wire	2:12	THIN THIGHS/TRANSIENT SQUATTER/TEENAGE SKANK
"NEAT NEAT NEAT," The Damned	2:40	SUPER LUNGE/BACNE/THUG
"THAT'S WHEN I REACH FOR MY REVOLVER," Mission of Burma	3:40	TRANSIENT SQUATTER/POGO/ROCK
"WILL ANYTHING HAPPEN," Blondie	2:55	IGGY'S PUNCH/GO-GO/ROCK
"WOW & FLUTTER," Stereolab	3:05	PLUNGER/SIDESWIPE/SLITS LEG LIFT
TOTAL RUNNING TIME:	38:13	(Close enough for rock 'n' roll)

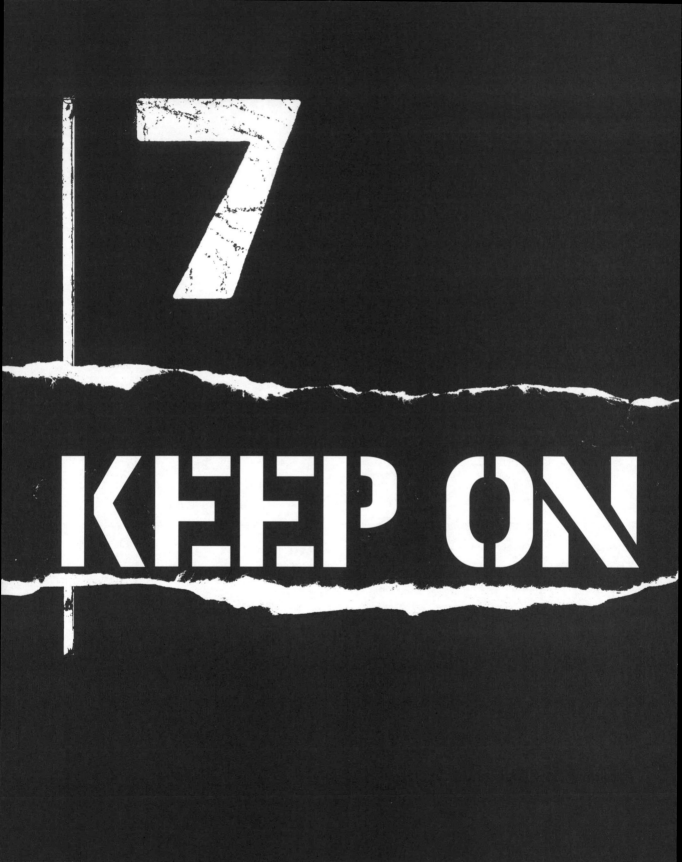

7

KEEP ON

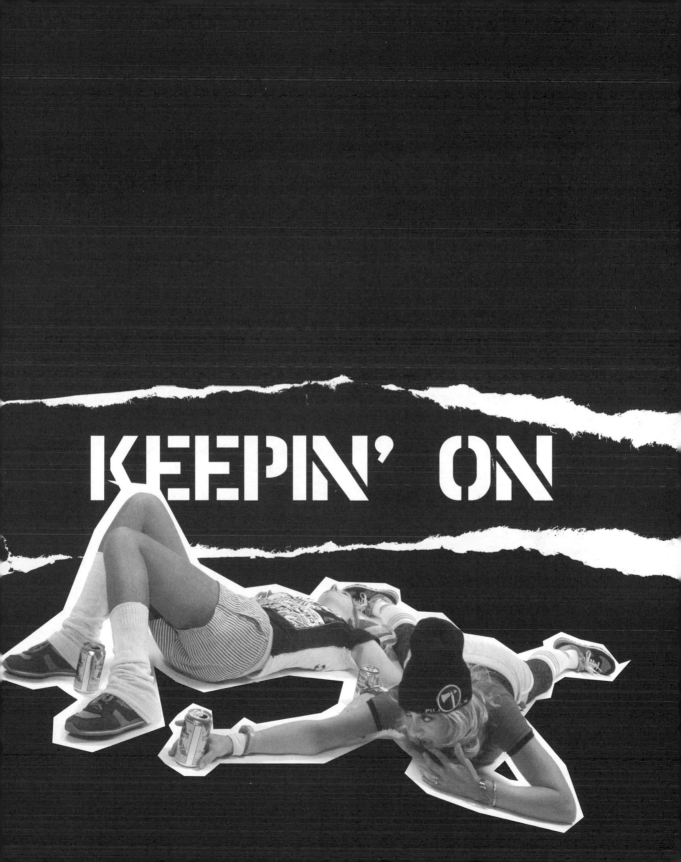

KEEPIN' ON

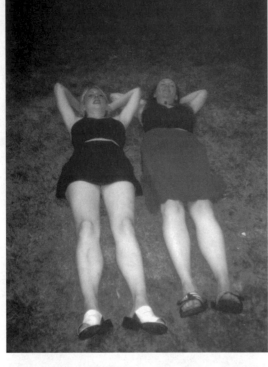

CRASH 'N' BURN:

HOW TO NOT BURN OUT ON YOUR WORKOUT

ONCE YOU MAKE IT through a few workouts, it's easy to get stoked. Getting started can be so hard that you may hardly believe you did it at all. You might get so psyched, you do it the next day—and even though you've already blown through a tin of Tiger Balm like a bond trader with a gram of coke late at the office, you still want to do it again. The more you exercise, the easier it gets, and you feel less awkward and more confident each time. You find yourself entertaining notions that once would have horrified you, such as riding your bike to work instead of driving or taking the train.

After about a week, you wonder when you might see some changes, even though you know that it's too soon. So you plug away, and soon begin to ask yourself when you can add more reps, or dream about getting through twenty minutes of cardio without feeling like you're about to collapse onto the nearest recliner. You feel like a champ and start imagining your face on a box of Wheaties. So *this* is what it felt like to be one of those happy athletic kids! You keep going and push harder, even though you feel like you might gag on your own vomit halfway through a couple of Roto-Rooters. After you're done, you feel like you were hit by a truck, but that doesn't stop you from doing it again the next day. You're unstoppable, a muscle car on the fast track to fitness … it's wiping you out, but this is good, right? Exercise is supposed to take the edge off, right? You start to feel a sense of dread before you begin your workout. There you are, standing in front of the stereo with the furniture shoved in a corner, dressed in your favorite ratty old Hüsker Dü shirt and a pair of shorts, goose pimples on your legs. Am I really about to do this again? Then you push Play, the music starts, and you go for it.

NOW THAT YOU'VE ROCKED hard and long enough to make it to the last chapter, a new question arises: If you decide that exercise is for you, what's going to happen between now and the point at which you achieve the desired state of health and discipline, to say nothing of the lasting status of Punk Rock Aerobics demigod? What are the good things you can expect to happen on the way, and what obstacles can you expect to confront? The test of your DIY philosophy is whether or not you can stick with what you've started. The least we can do is to sketch you a road map with big arrows pointing to the pitfalls. That way, maybe you won't get sucker punched by the same problems that knocked us on our flabby asses.

THEN ONE DAY you come home after your boss chews you out at work, or maybe you just feel crummy for no particular reason. All you want to do is chill, with no obligations. The idea of responsibility is so repulsive that you don't feel like being responsible toward yourself. That's cool, you've been working out a lot, and one day won't matter much. The next day you jump back into it and keep pretty regular for a week. Now it's been a couple of weeks, and you start to check yourself out in the mirror. Is anything changing? You wonder if it's working. Even though you've been sleeping better and feel good you want to see effects. Maybe you've been dieting and can step on the scale and see that you've lost a pound or two. But what if you haven't seen any changes? You've been working out like crazy! What's going on? Maybe you begin to get a little bored. Every day the same thing, jump up and down like a poodle at the circus, lift some weights, ho hum, yawn. Enough for now. This feels too hard today. You wonder why you don't have the energy for it. It looks as though your speeding Chevelle has run out of gas. Maybe you ought to throw a tarp over it and park it in the driveway for the winter.

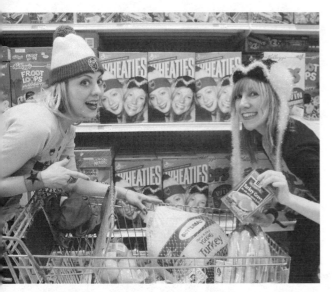

Delusions of grandeur

This is the *Behind the Music* approach to exercise. Live fast, die young. You were another doomed cliché trampled on the bumpy road to fitness. According to *Fitness for Dummies*, 50 percent of all new exercisers quit within the first eight weeks. Most of the people we know (including ourselves) were ready to drop out in the first eight minutes. Even now, we have days when we show up to teach our classes and hope that maybe we'll get lucky and nobody will show up. Then we could go home. Sometimes we feel lazy, or maybe one of us is feeling drained and just downed five extra-strength Midols. It's hard enough to jump up and down, but throw in all the screaming, and good god, if we aren't ready it's like taking our certification exams all over again. On the flipside, there are days when we show up and we're bouncing off the walls with the energy and stamina of the Energizer Bunny overdosed on ephedrine. We have a blast and it even feels easy at times. These are the moments that help us to keep it all in perspective. But one thing's for sure: as hard as it is to start exercising, it's even harder to keep going.

GET A GRIP ON YOURSELF
WE'RE LIKE A BROKEN RECORD on this point: when it comes to whether or not you exercise, the choice is yours alone to make. To do this with a sense of empowerment and control, it's important to know who you are and what you want from this decision. We're not asking you to go into the woods and meditate about this, *you just have to know you want to do it.*

DO IT FOR YOURSELF

WE MENTIONED earlier that it's punk to "do what you want and not give a rat's ass about what anyone else thinks." Now is the time to walk the talk. Exercise, like punk rock, is not about going through the motions because somebody else wants you to.

When you make up reasons to work out that you don't feel in your bones—even ones that seem legit—they usually crap out on you after a while. Wanting to be in better shape solely to impress the new guy in class or at work is only going to last as long as it takes for him to hook up with Sheila in the mailroom. At that point, you will feel defeated enough to watch TV and eat bags of Cheetos until the next solar eclipse. As dippy as it sounds, you need to ask yourself whether you want to get in shape for real, for yourself, and for no one else. Yes, we are having a Richard Simmons moment here, but let's run with it— "This is for you!" If you've ever tried to quit smoking, you know what we mean. Eventually, if your heart is in it, you can make it.

KNOW WHAT YOU WANT TO ACHIEVE BY ADOPTING AN EXERCISE PLAN

NOW'S THE TIME to think about what it is you hope to accomplish. Are you planning to try out for the lead when VH1 decides to make *The Iggy Pop Story*? Well, you're going to have your work cut out for you, ab master. Maybe you're hoping to take your mind off the fact that your girlfriend ran off with some idiot bass player with a mod haircut, and you want to build muscle so that you can kick his ass when he comes through town again. Maybe you want to lose weight and feel better about yourself. If you're doing it to fish for compliments, or keep up with your boyfriend who rides his bike everywhere, or to tone up and slim down for your fortieth birthday party, we don't care, and it doesn't matter. You don't have to turn figuring out why you're gonna get into shape into a freakin' therapy session— life is complicated enough. We just want to make sure you're clear about why you're doing it, because when it comes down to it, only you can find the inspiration to haul ass hyena.

YOU MIGHT SUPPRESS your gag reflex and try to come up with a mantra like one of the following. Don't worry, you don't have to write it down. In fact, it might be better if you don't leave any evidence.

"i wAnt to Do this BeCAuse i AM so stiFF i CAN't Bend oVer to LACe My Docs."

"I want to do this because I don't want to go insane from stress and anxiety."

"I want to do this because I am flabbier than a vat of Jell-O."

"I want to do this because I don't want to get stuck in front of the TV night after night because I feel bad about going out and people seeing how much weight I've gained."

"I WANT TO DO THIS because I just had a baby and I want to squeeze back into hot leather pants."

"I want to do this because when I hook up and get lucky some night, I don't want gettin' naked to be a humiliating experience."

"I WANT TO DO THIS TO BE ABLE TO TELL PEOPLE TO PISS OFF AND NOT LIVE IN FEAR OF A CRITICAL BEATDOWN."

"i WANt TO Do THIS so thAt i'LL Be iN Good enouGh shApe to teACh PunK rOCK AeroBics."

"I want to do this so that I'll look good in that dominatrix cat suit I got at a yard sale last week."

"I WANT TO DO THIS BECAUSE I WANT TO GET INTO SHAPE WITHOUT STARVING MYSELF"

"I want to do this because I look like a frumpy old lady right now and I'm not old enough for the sewing circle."

"I want to do this because I am going on tour and I'll be lucky if I can get through four songs without passing out."

"i wAnt to Do tHis BeCAusE i'M sicK OF It AlL."

KNOW YOUR PHYSICAL LIMITS, AND BE REALISTIC ABOUT THEM

HERE'S A DUMB THING TO DO: start working out like a jailbird in the weight room without seeing a doctor first. If you've been leading the life of a contentedly sedentary slack machine, you need to make sure that everything is cool before you throw your body into a state of shock. If you're fortunate enough to have health insurance, get a physical and let them know that you want to start working out. This is basic stuff. You wouldn't take your beater of a car cross-country without having it checked out first, would you? Okay, we know some of you would probably take a rusted-out school bus on a national tour without looking under the hood, but when the dashboard flies off outside Minneapolis, don't say we didn't warn you.

Since everything depends on your physical condition when you begin, your progress and the challenges you face will be different from those of others. You must take into account your age, weight, general health and level of fitness. If you're older, it will take longer to build muscle. If you're overweight, your body will have to work harder. If you are uncoordinated you need to give it time and get used to clearing fragile objects from your workout zone. If you have back problems you need to be extremely careful not to make them worse with an excess of enthusiasm and a deficit of technique. You have to work with the body you've got. You may have a lot of energy and even some muscle, but if you spent the past thousand nights listening to records and chugging Miller Lites, you might be in for a rough ride when you decide to rev up for your twenty-minute cardio rock block. If the physique of Iggy Pop is what you truly want, but you're working with the body of the white-jumpsuit Elvis (that the King was ever a karate champ is hard to believe, but we'll address physical deterioration later), it will require a lot of patience and determination.

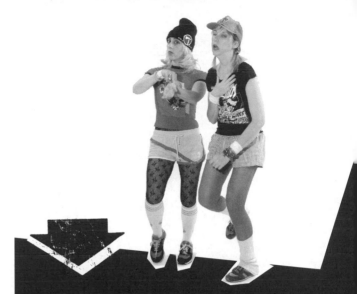

WHEN WE FIRST STARTED working out, we did so many things wrong that it's a wonder we stuck with it. The experience was also very different for each of us. For starters, our bodies are different. Hilken is shorter and she's got more T and A going on. Maura is long and boxy, with skinny arms and legs. There's a reason why our friend TD has nicknamed us Bitch Tits and Chicken Legs. Hilken has a background in dance. She was into ballet as a kid and studied at the Boston Conservatory after high school. She'd already been in good shape at one time in her life—really good shape. That all went down the tubes when she dropped out to play rock and roll, of course, but Maura had never been in shape, having lived in fear of all things sports-related. From head to toe, she was a preserve for virgin flab.

We trained together, doing the same cardio workout with the same weights at the same time. Within six weeks, Hilken's body began to change. She was less chubby and more statuesque. Her arms and shoulders had more definition. She also seemed to be losing weight, even though we weren't dieting. We were actually eating a lot more.

BUT THINGS WERE DIFFERENT for Maura, who at thirty-eight is the resident senior citizen. It was as though her body were saying, "Are you kidding? You must be messin' with me, so I'm just going to ignore you." After three months, she started to look more toned, but without muscle definition. Maura also started to feel an aching pain in the shin of her right leg. Repeating "no pain, no gain," over and over, she ignored it. One day while she was teaching class her leg got stiffer and stiffer, and the pain became much worse. She was prepared to keep biting her lip, but the next day she couldn't walk, so she went to the hospital. They took X-rays and found hairline stress fractures all over her right tibia. The injury was a classic case of too much too soon, Crash 'n' Burn syndrome; the bone hadn't built up enough density to tolerate all the jumping. It took two months of walking on crutches to heal. This is why we try to hammer home the point that you should see your doctor and know your limits. In the end, it took Maura six months of regular exercise to feel a marked improvement in strength and cardio endurance. It would be nice if the process of getting healthy were like a punk song—fast, balls out the whole time, two and a half minutes long. Guess what? It ain't.

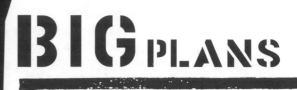

BIG PLANS

IT'S NOT ENOUGH to know what you want. You need to know how to get it. If you dive into aerobics without a strategy, you're setting yourself up to fail. You don't really think the Sex Pistols were an accident, do you? They were a well-crafted exercise in controlled chaos. They played formal gigs, worked the press, obtained and lost two record deals *and* got to keep the money. It wasn't called the Great Rock 'n' Roll Swindle for nothing. It required a plan, and a plan usually requires some goals.

Let's assume that you've got it all figured out. You smoke, drink, stay up late, and live on chips and Twinkies. Walking up a flight of stairs leaves your respiratory system in a shambles and you can't lift a two-liter bottle of Dr Pepper. You want to be able to mosh for more than five minutes without crashing to the floor like the Hindenburg. The next time you go to one of those shows, you want to be able to run around and have people jumping out of *your* way. You've checked yourself out in the mirror a million times and you've established that you're no Henry Rollins. You also lied to us and told us that you've seen a doctor and that everything is cool. So how are you going to do it?

SETTING GOALS

GOALS—THAT'S HOW. Having something to work toward helps. It will help you to understand what's down the pike and how far you've come. You need to set big dreamy goals, such as "I want to look more like Henry Rollins – Iggy Pop – Kim Gordon," in addition to humble short-term goals, such as "I will start lifting three-pound weights every other day." It might take you three years to meet your goal, but if it's broken down into smaller parts it'll be a lot less daunting.

LONG-TERM GOALS

THIS IS WHERE YOU GET TO THINK AHEAD. Drool over that pie in the sky. Be optimistic and ask for what you truly want. This can take three months, six months, or even a year, depending on what feels right to you. Whatever you choose, keep your goals reasonable with regard to the amount of time you give yourself. Obviously, if you are completely out of shape, it's going to take at least a year to bust out like a linebacker. Be as realistic as you can about the schedule.

"By this time next year, I want to be lifting twice as much weight and have no more flab."

"I will do my PRA workout for six months regularly and stay focused on strength training."

"In two years, I want to be buff enough to be a bouncer at a club."

"If it takes me six months to do this damn workout just once without collapsing, I will be stoked."

SHORT-TERM GOALS

WE LOVE THESE. They are the part of getting there that feels good, especially if you're the type who likes to write to-do lists and check off the items one at a time. Short-term goals are the ones you set just to get through the day or week or month. You can dream all you want about touring in stadiums with your band and churning out platinum records for RCA , but if you don't pick up your guitar and write some tunes, it's not going to happen. You need to barrel through a lot of little goals to make the big goals happen.

"By the end of the month I will switch from three-pound to five-pound weights."

"Each week this month, I am going to add five more reps to my ab work."

"Twice this week, I will try the full one-hour PRA workout."

"Every day, I will brush my teeth—dude, I've got like five left."

HERE'S HOW WE DID IT

In the beginning, our long-term goals were to get into good enough shape to pass the infernal certification exam, and ultimately to be able to teach the class. The latter turned out to be much harder. We needed to be in good enough shape to survive the workout, scream and yell, pay attention to the class, maintain our technique, get over our stage fright, and at least look as if we were having fun.

With the goal of passing the exam, we began working out four times a week to whatever aerobics video we had on hand. After a couple of weeks we incorporated weights and floor exercises and they thrashed us so hard that we never again worked out without them. While we were doing this, we developed our own routine, and after about six weeks we switched to our own insane workout. It was harder but more fun. We continued to make the floor and weight exercises harder and more challenging. Every week, we added on another ten crunches. Even if we couldn't get through them, we tried. If we heard or read about a new exercise for triceps, we tested it. If we were sore from the exercise, we were stoked that it had worked and tried it again.

FROM APATHY

CONTRARY TO WHAT WE BELIEVED, you don't need to be in tip-top shape to pass the certification exam for aerobics instructors. You do, however, need to be in decent shape and able to understand and demonstrate proper technique. Teaching the class really keeps a fire under our butts. When you've taken $7 apiece from twenty people who want to work out, you don't inform them that you have a headache and go home—you get up there and try to kick ass as hard as you can. After two years, we can handle the classes, but both of us still have exercises to work on. And, of course, we make ever loftier goals for ourselves. At the rate we're going, if we wanted to, we could be Navy SEALs next year.

Where are we now? Neither one of us is a mass of rippling muscles, but we never set out to be and we never cared to be. But we're bigger fitness tools than anybody who used to know us in our smoking days could imagine. After realizing that she didn't want to ride her bike through another Boston winter, Maura broke down and joined a gym so that she could continue getting a cardio workout when she wasn't doing PRA. For the first two months, she donned a wig and sunglasses so that she wouldn't be spotted watching VH1 Stories and Legends while going nuts on the treadmill. Hilken has been caught using her natural flexibility to get dirty with Downward Dog, sweating it out in the 100-degree heat of a Power Yoga class. We've reverse-aged from frail youths to robust, pink-cheeked grown-ups.

WHAT IF NONE OF THIS WORKS? What if you just want to quit? Brace yourself for the possibility. The chances that you will want to quit are high. If you've spent your life as a nonexerciser, they are even higher. According to the handy textbook that we purchased from the Aerobics and Fitness Association of America to study for our exam, the main reasons for not wanting to begin or continue an exercise program are time, willpower, and apathy—and we know that you guys are probably world authorities on all three of them.

TO ATROPHY

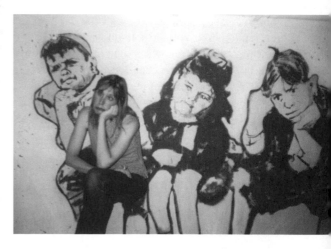

"Ho-hum."

NO TIME

SO YOU'RE FEELING APATHETIC. *Boo hoo.* We don't feel sorry for you at all, but since we've written this book and are trying to help you out, we'll address it. Few things are as funny or as pathetic in life as people just not giving a shit. Why don't you get your "Please Kill Me" T-shirt out of the closet and walk through Times Square. I doubt anyone would even notice, and if they did, they certainly wouldn't be concerned about it. Too bad. True apathy is a serious sign of depression—a problem that demands medical attention; the kind of apathy that prevents people from exercising is usually grounded in bunk philosophy, laziness, or fear.

Pull yourself together, kid. Feeling apathetic about exercise is good for only one thing, and that is the multitude of lamebrain excuses it tends to produce. People who "just don't feel like it" come up with some of the best reasons of all not to exercise.

"The dog ate my mat."

"My tattoos are healing and I can't move around too much."

"I have athlete's foot."

"I'll just have a lot of sex instead."

"I don't need to. My mom was always skinny and she never lifted a finger."

"Men like big butts."

"It's cooler to drink and smoke butts than care about your health."

"I'm not vain enough to exercise."

"I don't want to live after thirty-five anyway."

Give us a break.

LET'S MOVE ON to a more practical, grown-up problem (we know there are practical grown-ups among you)—time. It's limited, and it's valuable. We all understand what it is to have no time. In this day and age, you can barely pay your rent without working your full-time job along with another crappy part-time job ... unless you're doing something illegal, or you're in computers, investing, or pharmaceuticals. If you're an artist or musician type, let's face it: you are screwed in this department. You'll be lucky if you get any time to squeeze in some regular band practice, or work on that diorama made out of animal bones and burned toothpicks.

There's no way around this one—you have to make time. Don't tell us that you don't know how. If you've ever been pursued by bill collectors (especially the ones that descend on you for unpaid student loans), you know that they don't take no for an answer. They know that you must be spending at least $30 a week on something that you can live without, whether it's a new CD, a few beers, or cable television. If you think that you don't have time, think again; there has got to be something useless you waste it on. Think of how much time you squander on the phone, talking to people whom you wish never had your phone number in the first place, or how often you cruise the Internet looking up info on some obscure band, scoping out prices on eBay, or hanging in some weirdo chat room talking about nothing at all. The truth is, most of us find a little time somewhere in our schedules when there is something we *really* want to do.

The amount of time that you need to spend on a workout for it to make a difference is much less than you think. We've heard everything from ten minutes a day to thirty minutes a day, but probably it's safe to say that if you're starting up for the first time, twenty minutes of cardio every other day will get the job done. Add ten minutes of weights on off days and you'll really be keeping death at bay. If you can find a small gap in your

P.R.A. GOES TO THE MOVIES

IF YOU'RE THE RIGHT AGE, you might remember the night your parents took you to The Karate Kid and you wouldn't stop throwing jump kicks in your bedroom until they force-fed you warm milk and dragged you into bed at two in the morning. Why not apply that experience to your quest for fitness? Here are ten punk rock flicks that will get you in the mood to rock yesterday's burger into oblivion.

ROCK 'N' ROLL HIGH SCHOOL (1979)
With the help of the Ramones, a gang of rebellious students seizes control of their high school from a rock 'n' roll-hating administration. Inspirational scene: Watchin' the school burn, baby, burn.

TIMES SQUARE (1980)
Two teenage girls from different backgrounds run away from a mental hospital, steal an ambulance, and start a punk band called the Sleez Sisters. Inspirational scene: The performance on the Times Square marquee.

THE DECLINE OF WESTERN CIVILIZATION
(Documentary, 1981)
Penelope Spheeris's camera travels through the vital organs of the early L.A. punk scene, from zine editorial offices to illegal living spaces. Inspirational scene: Darby Crash of the Germs musters more energy onstage then any athlete we've ever seen, and the best part is that he's too wasted to remember his own made-up name.

REPO MAN (1984)
A disgruntled punk rock weirdo gets a job repossessing cars after losing his grocery store job. He stumbles into a surreal world of conspiracy theories, major freaks, and cosmic intrigue. Inspirational scene: A repossessed Malibu makes an unplanned trip to outer space.

ANOTHER STATE OF MIND
(Documentary, 1984)
It's the early eighties, and two SoCal punk bands, Social Distortion and Youth Brigade, hit the road to play any grime-encrusted venue that will have them. Inspirational scene: The boys push the dead school bus cum tour van through Washington, D.C., in a historic fusion of punk and strength training.

SUBURBIA a.k.a. THE WILD SIDE (1983)
Drama about runaway SoCal punk rock kids squatting in an abandoned house in the suburbs written and directed by Penelope Spheeris, who gave us The Decline of Western Civilization and Wayne's World. Inspirational scene: The troubled youngsters rock themselves silly at shows.

SID & NANCY (1986)
A young actor by the name of Gary Oldman is pitch perfect as Sid Vicious, the incompetent but legendary Sex Pistols bassist, who remains somehow endearing despite descending into the misery of heroin addiction and stabbing the attention-craving love of his life, Nancy Spungen. Directed by Alex Cox, also responsible for Repo Man. Inspirational scene: Oldman head-bangs like a gorilla at a concert attended by a mohawked infant.

1991: THE YEAR PUNK BROKE
(Documentary, 1992)
Nirvana, Sonic Youth, Dinosaur Jr., and other bands approaching their peak popularity tour Europe at the dawn of grunge. Inspirational scene: Kurt Cobain, still an obscure singer, runs in circles and flops around on the stage like a wounded insect. Floor exercise, redefined.

THE FILTH AND THE FURY
(Documentary, 2000)
The story of the Sex Pistols told from the perspective of the now prosperous and middle-aged extant band members. None of them have a kind word for Malcolm MacLaren, the Svengali who made them stars, but the music backs up their insistence that they were first and foremost a rock 'n' roll band, not Malc's freak show. Inspirational scene: A little kid bounces like a happy rabbit at the Pistols' benefit concert for laid-off firefighters.

24-HOUR PARTY PEOPLE (2002)
A history of Manchester's Factory Records, the music label that nurtured the career of the seminal band Joy Division. Inspirational scene: The Sex Pistols play their first show in Manchester, and the local rock crowd, still clad in early seventies hippie regalia, catches the vibe and spontaneously begins to pogo.

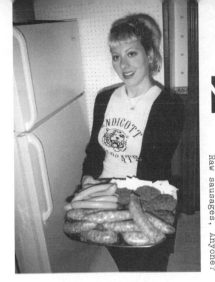

Raw sausages, Anyone?

NO WILLPOWER

WHAT IF you care about the state of your body, but improving it seems too hard? You despair at the shape you're in now. You've gone so far as to buy a couple of videos to get started, but you end up watching them from the La-Z-Boy with a bucket of popcorn in your lap, offering fashion advice to the instructor. Then you Fast-Forward to see how hard the moves are. After the credits roll, you go back to the beginning and watch again, as if repeated viewings were almost as good as exercise. Lack of willpower is when you know you should try—and even want to try—but for some reason, you don't have the battery power to get up and running.

Here are some tips to help you find your inner track star and conquer your lack of willpower:

day to work out regularly, use it. If you wake up or come home at the same times every day, it should be easy. When we first began working out at home, we would wake up half an hour earlier to fit it into our daily torture. After about three weeks, things didn't feel right if we skipped the workout to sleep longer. It becomes part of what you do, the same way you might eat dinner at a certain hour every night. Remember, it's better to spend some time on exercise than none at all. Lots of people spend a lot of time working out, but that's because the more you do it, the more you like it. You actually want to devote time to those Super Lunges and bricks, or just zipping around on your bike.

• Work with the short-term goals outlined here. You won't be paralyzed if you try to do a small thing every two days. If you're laboring desperately under sky-high standards, you'll succumb to the lure of the couch.

• Make it easy on yourself. Keep your workout short and sweet in the beginning, and reward yourself when you're done. An ice-cold Pabst and a cheeseburger, a bottle of wine, or a box of chocolates—you decide.

• Ask yourself if sitting around measuring your spare tire will make you feel more fit.

• Remind yourself of how great you will feel if you try at all—like the high you feel after a great rock concert.

• Sometimes you have to try and try again until the routine sticks—how many times did Uncle Ned try to give up Lucky Strikes before you stopped smelling them on his breath? Don't give up. You know you can do it eventually; you just can't do it with your ass sewn to the chair.

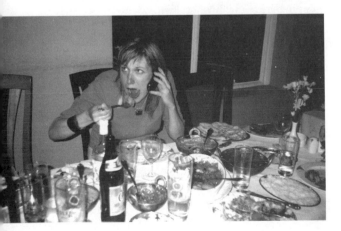

I want to call in another order
of chicken vindaloo!

WHAT HAPPENED? What hit you? How come all of a sudden you feel like a wet sand castle, getting softer by the minute? You started off so strong. You were wicked hardcore. You were the king of crunches. Your abdomen was like the north face of the Grand Canyon. But little by little, your exercise routine tapered into nothing, and you're not sure why. Maybe you're suffering from crash 'n' burn; maybe you got bored. You're not sure, but for whatever reason, your victory march ground to a halt. Maybe when you first started reading this book, you were more motivated than you are now. You may be thinking, *Why forge ahead? What's the point? How do I know I'll stick with this? I'm a born quitter. Damn it, there was a reason I was always got picked last for kickball—the other kids took one look at me and knew I was doomed. It is downright natural that I should spend the rest of my days wasting away with a Blockbuster Video membership to keep me company.*

Sometimes you don't even intend to quit, it just happens. Maybe you were doing great before you picked up West Nile virus camping at an outdoor music festival. The next thing you know, you're committed to a hospital bed for three weeks and the result of all your hard work went goes down the toilet. Or the distraction is you took a vacation in Venice (who wants to exercise on vacation anyway?), and you just can't do jumping jacks in your hotel when you can see the canals from your window. It happens. All of us have moments when we let down our guard, when life throws a wrench in our plans.

If you seriously doubt that you can get back on the treadmill of rock, just remember: one or two days a week are better than none. Don't blame yourself for feeling like a quitter. You may have cold feet because you're starting something new. It's normal to pull back from new experiences. You need to try to keep working out. If you've been doing this and want to take a break, it's cool. It's not the end of the world; on the other hand, you need to know what happens when you do.

DECAY

THERE'S NO ACTION: LOSING AND REGAINING MUSCLE

SO HOW LONG does it take to fall out of shape and revert to your old mushroom-textured self? Not long; it doesn't matter how long you've been at it, either. When it comes to aerobic fitness, this can happen as quickly as two weeks. To stop working out entirely isn't the end of the world, but you can't expect to jump back in the game without a fight (see sidebar).

RECENTLY, we took our classes to the U.K., where we put on a demonstration for extreme sports dudes at a skateboarding and music festival. We'd hardly finished a stint of classes in New York and we were exhausted and our schedules were inhumane. At a certain point, we lost our grip on our own workout routines—we were only working out when we had classes. When we finally got to back to Massachusetts and realized that we had to jump back into the Boston class, it had been a couple of weeks since we'd done the full workout. We were in dire straits. We got up there and gagged our way through the routine. We were a disgrace to Punk Rock Aerobics. Half the class could've kicked our asses inside out. Take this advice: don't get too cocky about your fitness. The gains you make are fleeting if you don't work to maintain them.

But here's what you can learn from this particular instance of stupidity: try not to stop altogether. Instead of using our downtime to scarf fish 'n' chips and a few pints at the pub, we should have taken our own advice and put aside fifteen minutes every other day to run around Hyde Park. When it comes to cardio, even getting through half of your regular routine makes a difference.

THE GOOD NEWS: once you stop working out, it takes as long as you spent building muscle to lose what you gained, but only one-third of that time to get the muscles back. So if you blow off a week or two, it doesn't' mean that you'll be a jelly donut with legs. Your muscles won't turn into fat like a pumpkin into a carriage. There's payback for all the work you've done.

When you try to bounce back after your break, it may take a week or even three before you stop feeling sore; but if you stop for a week or two every time you feel sore, you'll have to go through that soreness each time, as if it were brand new. Why would you want to relive the trauma an infinite number of times, like Bill Murray in *Groundhog Day*? If you keep going that way, you'll eventually surrender to the pain. So bite the bullet and work your way through the soreness, soldier. You'll thank yourself for it later.

If you find that you're getting burned out on this workout, cut loose and take a week off. Or try some different variations offered at the end of Chapter 6. And don't punish yourself by using the same song over and over or otherwise bleeding the fun out of your routine. Once your body gets used to moving again and you find a way to keep your brain entertained, you'll be craving more. Trust us—we've probably been as unfit as you are now, no matter how slothful you are.

FITNESS FOR YOUR TOILET

Gray instructional photos and lots of preachy instruction are a recipe for boredom—perfect for bathroom reading.

FITNESS FOR DUMMIES. Informative, accessible, and demystifying. If you're looking for a second fitness book, we recommend this one.

DEFINITION, by Joyce L. Vedral. We bought this book in a thrift store thinking it'd be good for cheap laughs. It is one of the finest books we own. Joyce is a fitness expert who earned a doctorate in English and psychology from New York University. She claims that the only reason she got into fitness is because "being out of shape was draining my energy and stealing my creativity." Her books are among the best-written and least intimidating fitness books we've seen, and also among the funniest. We love Joyce because she's a smart lady who knows how to laugh at herself.

JANE FONDA'S WORKOUT BOOK. You gotta hand it to Jane: somehow she manages to maintain her feminist, politically correct stance without being as heavy-handed as you'd expect. Moreover, her song choices are worth their weight in gold. A sampler: "Souvenirs" by Dan Fogelberg, "I Love a Rainy Night" by Eddie Rabbit, "I Will Survive" by Gloria Gaynor.

RICHARD SIMMONS' NEVER GIVE UP: INSPIRATIONS, REFLECTIONS, STORIES OF HOPE, by Richard Simmons: They don't call the man "the pied piper of fitness" for nothing. We love Richard. As the story goes, he was a 300-pound out-of-work actor who one day found a note on his windshield that read, "Fat people die young, please don't die." He had a distinguished career before he became a fitness guru, having been an extra in the infamous party scene in Fellini's SATYRICON. Read anything by Richard. He knows what it means to be an outsider—and what it means to be a true original.

WHAT HAPPENS IF YOU STOP WORKING OUT FOR A MONTH OR TWO AND YOU'RE STILL NOT READY FOR A COMEBACK?

REMEMBER HOW when we first started working out together, Hilken, the former ballet dancer, started to get buff long before Maura showed any sign of building muscle? That's a perfect example of how your body retains some memory of its old condition, even if you've been letting it crumble for years. So keep in mind that even if you spent many months sedentary, you'll bounce back even if you make half the effort that you put in when you were suffering on the mat for the first time.

In *Definition*, the *Anna Karenina* of aerobics literature, Joyce Vedral writes:

```
Did you know that women lose about 1 percent
of bone mass a year after they turn 35?
And now they are saying that this bone loss
doubles after menopause. The good news is:
you can gain the bone mass you've lost by
working out. Bones grow in response to work-
ing your muscle mass. Your muscles grow in
response to being forced to work.
```

Let's take a moment to contemplate the sweetness Dr. Vedral has spelled out for us: all you have to do is work your muscles to add bone mass as well as muscle. So even if you can't get inspired by the progress you see in the mirror, keep in mind that when you work out, a lot of the benefits are invisible. Putting the screws on your muscles could keep your skeleton from crumbling long after your moshing days are over. So don't depend solely on changes in the way you look. Think about how much you like walking without a cane.

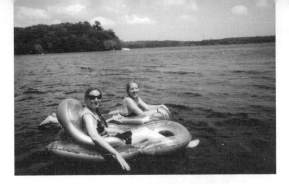

Three years ago this was our idea of swimming.

SICK OF US?

WE WOULD BE THRILLED to think that you started your PRA workout and felt that you couldn't live without it, that it laid waste to all fitness alternatives; but we seriously doubt this to be the case. If you get into better shape you may want to try some other things with your newfound confidence. One of the best ways to keep fitness a part of your life is to strive to make it new. Branch out into the unknown. Try something different, even if it's just a brand-new mix. If you get bored, don't come crying to us, do something about it. See the world.

Terrible to confess, Punk Rock Aerobics isn't the only weird workout out there. We hear about all kinds of things that sound at least marginally fun (well, fun to us, now that we've gotten over our fear of fitness). At some point, you might want to take the party out of your living room and start to experiment a little. Maybe you want to try out belly dancing or Go-Go Aerobics—we strongly suspect that the music may not suck. Maybe your neighborhood is tough enough to make karate or even boxing a practical life skill—you could add technique to newfound brawn. Classes can be great because no matter how much you hated team projects in chemistry, sometimes you work harder in a group. When you feel as though you're about to quit, you can't because you'll feel like too much of a pussy if you walk out in the middle!

LET'S TAKE THIS OUTSIDE

IF YOU PREFER the open air to the gym, don't worry: you'll never exhaust the planet's capacity to put the human body through the wringer. We love riding bikes instead of driving, and if you're more ambitious than we are, you can attack hills. If you don't have a bike, check out your local Goodwill or comb through yard sales. You can find one for $50 or less, and it is worth every penny. Bicycles are cheap, fun, and you never have to worry about parking. Just do your skull a favor and wear a helmet.

Here's a new one for you—start walking. It's unbelievable how many people drive short distances out of habit. Walking is something you can do anywhere, whether you live in the most congested block in Queens or the loneliest corner of the Mojave. Walking only twenty minutes every few days will do almost as much to improve your fitness as a full workout. Get a dog if you need more motivation. Once you have a dog, regular walking quickly becomes the most attractive of your options.

If you're lucky enough to be near water, swim. Public pools may gross you out, but most have enough germ-killing chlorine to blind you for a week and turn your hair green. Some pools are more sanitary and chemical-free than others, but you need to do some research to find them. If you live near a lake or the beach, you have no excuse at all.

We also know that some of you are closet trustfunders, so don't be ashamed to revert back to your childhood affection for archery, golf, and horseback riding. Even in New York City you can go to the park and get on a horse. Rent a canoe with your friends, go ice-skating, or start gardening. Hell, take up polo. We won't tell your homeless friends.

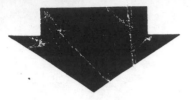

GETTING

GANGS OF NEW YORK
Classic New York hardcore bands, according to AMERICAN HARDCORE, by Steven Blush:

- Cro-Mags
- Murphy's Law
- Agnostic Front
- Youth of Today

P.R.A. Q&A #11

JD Samson
Le Tigre

If you exercise, what type of exercise do you do? And what kind of music do you listen to when working out?

I run, ride my bike and lift weights. I listen to whatever is playing in the gym: hip-hop and house.

What songs or records have inspired you to physically move?

Yaz, Sean Paul.

Do you like your body, or are you among the ranks of people who think that if they could just lose those ten pounds, they'd be perfect?

I think I could lose in a few areas. But I think it's ok. I want to be chiseled.

Is skinny better than buff?

No way.

Johanna Fateman
Le Tigre

Has your state of "being in shape" ever affected your performance either positively or negatively? Do you tend to work up a sweat onstage?

I sweat a lot onstage and it definitely helps my performance if I have been able to workout in the weeks before tour. Cardiovascular strength is important to be able to jump around and freak out but still have some control over vocal performance.

As a performer in the public eye, has body image ever been a concern? Have you ever had outside pressure (that is, from a label, etc.) about your weight/shape?

Obviously there is a ton of cultural pressure for women to be super thin. I try not to let it get me down cuz I know in my heart that being healthy and sexy is not about that.

HOOKED

WHEN WE FIRST started this whole exercise thing, we felt that we'd never get used to it. We were sore all the time, getting injured, and getting hate mail. We had to ask ourselves, is exercise paying off?

Yet slowly, we began to understand that the reason we stuck to it was that we were getting hooked. The fact that exercise was starting to feel good was something we could not ignore. Sure, running into people and getting compliments helped. Maura would bump into people who'd barely recognized her (even though she did chop off twelve inches of hair). Gradually it crept up on us that exercise was our way of life and we didn't want to stop.

Maura suddenly was riding her bike everywhere. Hilken started taking yoga classes and trying out every new exercise in *Shape* magazine. We went jogging around a pond that we could once barely motivate ourselves to walk around. When we went swimming, we would really swim, as opposed to floating around like cadavers. The ugly truth is that we had become people who liked to exercise—we didn't want to stop for too long or take a week off. It actually made us a little bit crazy if we did. It's as though our bodies had their own agenda and needed us to take care of them. They made us want to keep doing the PRA workout, ride our bikes, and dance all night to bad eighties music. We might as well cop to it: we made fitness something we want to do for the rest of our f@#%ed-up lives.

Believe it or not, once you've gotten used to it, your body will cry out for exercise. We're not saying Punk Rock Aerobics in particular will have you hooked—just that if you stick with this for six months, you will crave and desire some kind of activity. You may even come to consider this a sound state of mind, not a strange fitness culture malady.

P.R.A. Q&A #12

Paul Leary
Guiter Player for Butthole Surfers

....

Does Mike Watts cycling regime make you want to go out and buy a bike?

Just hearing the name "Mike Watt" makes me want to ride my bike ... to the cigar store.

Do you have a gym membership?

No, I heard my friends complain too much about the number of stairs they had to climb in the parking garage to get to their gym.

Have you ever pushed away the coffee table to dance until all hours of the morning?

Oh, ya. And in the nude, too. The music of Glenn Miller has that effect on me.

What songs or records have inspired you to physically move?

L7 used to make me violent. Now its the Donnas.

Do you tend to work up a sweat onstage?

Let me put it this way, if I need to pee real bad before hitting the stage but don't have time, it doesn't matter. I sweat it out. Peeing is for pussies.

What are your thoughts on Henry Rollins?

ABC Sports should hire Henry to do color commentary on Monday Night Football.

MINOR SWEAT

Your body wants to be used. You don't need to be doing something big. It adds up when you make small choices to lift, walk, and use stairs when you could pay for a service or use a machine. Fidgeters are said to burn up to 400 more calories a day than nonfidgeters. True or not, it does go some way in explaining how skinny everybody is in New York City. There's nothing wrong with pacing and chewing gum. Just keep moving.

Every chance you can, use the stairs, not escalators and elevators. If you have two bags of groceries and it's 90 degrees out, you shouldn't walk up six flights if you don't have to, but maybe you should walk up three and then take the elevator. Some people might think you're losing it, but we'd think you're a fitness stud if you take the stairs all the way.

The grocery store—the very den of sin where you might indulge a passion for Bud and Fritos—can be your best friend. Fill up the bags and carry them to your car your own damn self. Or even better, lug them home. It's free and it works.

Help your itinerant friends move. It's a great workout, besides being a nice thing to do. They will owe you so big-time that you can call them the next time you lose your job or get arrested.

And while you're at it, clean up that disgraceful rubbish bin you live in. Get down on your hands and knees and scrub. You'd be surprised what a good workout you can get from housework, and it will help you win the war against athlete's foot. You're not some kind of Stepford wife if you're doing it for yourself. And if you are a rocker, think about it this way: no matter what you might have thought in high school, there's nothing inherently punk about dirt. Paying a servant to clean up after you or leaving the job to your roommates isn't very DIY.

LAST RITES

WE KNOW that when you picked up this book you probably thought it would be fun—but fun relative to *Abs of Steel* or some other *Full Metal Jacket* approach to fitness that would have you on the floor counting like a robot for however long it took to break down and swear to never exercise again. Well, we hope Punk Rock Aerobics *is* fun. It is for us. If it weren't, we would have thrown in the sweaty towel ourselves by now. Let's face it, sometimes we can't keep a straight face looking at our own moves or better yet, when an entire section of the workout gets botched in the middle. Whatever it took to distract us and make us feel rewarded for our efforts, we did. After our Monday classes, the next stop is always cocktails and burgers. To go home to a plate of steamed broccoli after all that hard work would suck. What's the point of exercise, if not to give yourself some wiggle room where good behavior is concerned?

When it comes to having fun, pursue any means necessary. Find a friend to work out with, or do PRA at home with the whole posse. Play the songs you like and turn it into a hoe-down. Don't worry whether you're doing it "right." If your workout degenerates into a free-for-all danceathon in your living room, is that a bad thing? If you are moving and having fun doing it, you're on the right track. That's what it's all about.

If because of PRA just one sofa junkie starts riding a bike or walking, or if one embittered outcast from PE starts to think of PRA as preferable to Chinese water torture, our labors have not been in vain and we are stoked. We'd like it even better if you were inspired enough to do what we did and start your own class, your own way: Soft Porn Aerobics? Feel free to send us cash. The point is, you don't have to accept what's already out there or let it stop you from making your own path to fitness. The greatest victory for us would be if you decided you didn't need us anymore because you're too busy having fun your own way.

— HILKEN + MAURA

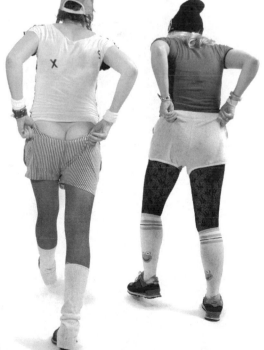

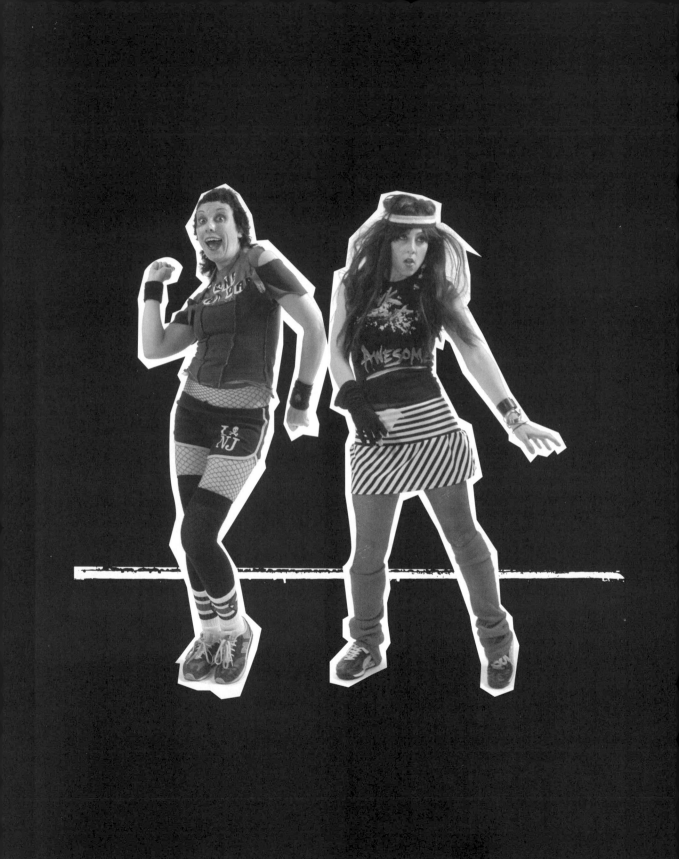

P.R.A. DISCOGRAPHY

HERE IT IS—PUNK ROCK 101. For those of you who might be checking out punk rock for the first time, here is a list of some classic records from the early days. We decided to keep to the basics: things that we like a lot and that we know will be fun in your **PRA** workout. It's not all classic punk; some could easily fall into another genre such as pop-punk. Also, most of the choices listed have been reissued on CD, so you should be able to buy them online or at your local indie shop. If you are a music snob, turn back now—you probably have this stuff, and you'll likely slam us for not including that obscure Rudimentary Peni record. We all have to start somewhere.

1. The Adverts *Crossing the Red Sea*, 1978 (Bright). Find out why Gaye Advert was one of the coolest women in punk.

2. The Avengers *The Avengers*, 1983 (CD Presents, Ltd.). You need to hear "Amerikan in Me" right now ("ask not what you can do for your country...but what your country's doin' for you"). There are some amazing pop hits on this record great for your PRA workout. Penelope Houston's vocals are punk, and so is her hairdo on the cover.

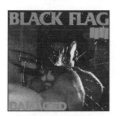

3. Black Flag *Damaged*, 1981 (SST). One of the best and most essential punk rock albums ever. Own it.

4. Blondie *Parallel Lines*, 1978 (Chrysalis). Okay, we know you don't think it's punk rock. Read *Making Tracks* and then talk to us. Deborah Harry was there at the beginning. And she is totally punk, in every way. Besides, Iggy thought so—and it's really easy to use one of these songs in your workout.

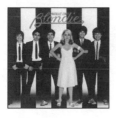

5. Buzzcocks *Singles Going Steady*, 1979 (IRS); *A Different Kind of Tension*, 1979 (IRS). Anything by this band is great in a PRA workout. Their songs are quick, perfect, and classic punk pop tunes.

6. The Clash *The Clash*, 1977 (Epic); *Give 'Em Enough Rope*, 1977 (Epic); *London Calling*, 1979 (Columbia). Perfect for pogoing.

7. The Cramps *Songs The Lord Taught Us*, 1980 (Illegal). Punk rock psychobilly. Poison Ivy is so hot—one of the first girl punk instrumentalists. Let Poison Ivy be your inspiration as you become a punk rock goddess.

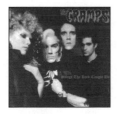

8. The Cure *Boys Don't Cry*, 1980 (Elektra/Asylum). You can tell us that this isn't punk, but we don't care. It's a classic, and Robert Smith is like a Gothic Elvis with his big hair and black mascara. It has the greatest dance songs on it.

9. The Damned *The Black Album*, 1980 (Chiswick).

10. Dead Boys *Young Loud and Snotty*, 1977 (Sire). Stiv Bators (deceased) is one of the punk rock legends of all time, with the classic song "Sonic Reducer." Practically every punk band has covered it. Never forget: Stiv is Sex.

11. The Descendents *Milo Goes to College*, 1982 (SST).

12. Devo *Q: Are We Not Men? A: We Are Devo*, 1978 (Warner Bros.). "Uncontrollable Urge" and "Jocko Homo" are some of the great songs on this one. Produced by Brian Eno.

13. The Fall *Live at the Witch Trials*, 1979 (Step Forward); *Hex Enduction Hour*, 1982 (Kamera); *The Wonderful and Frightening World of The Fall*, 1984 (Beggar's Banquet). Mark E. Smith is a talent not to be rivaled; get anything by The Fall.

14. Fear *The Record*, 1982 (Slash). "Let's Have a War" and "I Love Livin' in the City" are classic American punk anthems. Great record.

15. Gang of Four *Entertainment*, 1979 (EMI International). Import only. The classic hit "Damaged Goods" is on this one, and also the amazing song "Anthrax." (See rad interview with drummer Hugo Burnham on page 73).

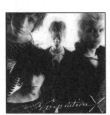

16. Generation X *Generation X*, 1978 (Chrysalis). Something of quality from Billy Idol.

17. The Germs *M.I.A.: The Complete Anthology*, 1979 (Slash). Darby was a tragic punk rock figure, like so many of the greats. How cool that this record was produced by Joan Jett.

18. Gun Club *Fire of Love*, 1981 (Ruby). Classic first Gun Club album; could describe it as punk blues. Good for stretches.

19. Hüsker Dü *Metal Circus*, 1983 (SST). "It's Not Funny Anymore" is such a great sad song. This album is a classic.

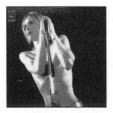

20. Iggy & The Stooges *Raw Power*, 1973 (CBS). This seminal record has so many great songs to inspire you for your workout: "Search and Destroy," "Raw Power"—you name it. Any Stooges or Iggy Pop record you can get your hands on (for example, *Fun House* or *Lust for Life*) is a must have. You can't go wrong— Iggy is Dog.

21. Joy Division *Unknown Pleasures*, 1979 (Warner Bros.). See where Interpol got their stuff . . . and if you can get your hands on any live footage of this band, you will be mesmerized and possibly understand the reason why Ian Curtis killed himself at such a young age. The only bummer is that their hit "Love Will Tear Us Apart" is not on this record and you have to hear that song on *The Peel Sessions*, 1993 (D.E.I). P.S. Find out how Tommy Shaw from Styx is involved with Joy Division. It'll make you puke.

22. Magazine *Real Life*, 1978 (Virgin). Howard Devoto left the Buzzcocks and made this great record. "Shot By Both Sides" is the hit.

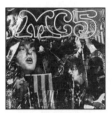

23. MC5 *Kick Out the Jams*, 1968 (Elektra). The first politically charged rock with a reason; one of the first records that pointed out the ills of society. Basically, more was going on in this record than "I Wanna Hold Your Hand"—not to mention that it's a rockin' album and a total dance move inspiration charger.

24. Minor Threat *Out of Step*, 1983 (Dischord). One of the greatest punk rock records. Features Ian Mackaye from Teen Idles and now of Fugazi.

25. The Minutemen *Buzz or Howl Under the Influence of Heat*, 1983 (SST). The songs "Cut" and "Little Man with a Gun in His Hand" are so great. Get this record for these songs alone: they are intricate and experimental but sharp and short. Plus, Mike Watt is one of our favorite legendary punk rockers.

26. The Misfits *Walk Among Us*, 1982 (Slash). You have to listen to this record to know what punk truly is. "Hatebreeders" and "I Turned into a Martian" are classics. Listen to it over and over. You won't get bored and you'll want to pogo to Danzig's madman vocals until you drop.

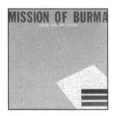

27. Mission of Burma *Signals, Calls, and Marches*, 1981 (Ace of Hearts); and *Vs.*, 1982 (Ace of Hearts). You must go out and buy both records now. They wrote incredible songs that are innovative to this day. "That's When I Reach for My Revolver" and "Academy Fight Song" are great pop songs to add to your work-out. We love them.

28. The Modern Lovers *The Modern Lovers*, 1976 (Beserkly). This is Jonathan Richman at his best. Early on, John Felice from The Real Kids was in the band (only for a moment).

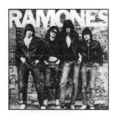

29. The Ramones *Ramones*, 1977 (Sire); *Rocket to Russia*, 1977 (Sire). A sure bet, just stick to the early years. Great for any PRA rock block!

30. The Replacements *Hootenanny*, 1983 (TwinTone). So many great songs on this one: "Run It," "Take Me Down to the Hospital"...really DIY, all the way.

31. The Rezillos *Can't Stand the Rezillos*, 1978 (Sire). Fun pop all the way.

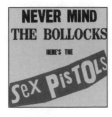

32. The Runaways *The Runaways*, 1976 (Polygram). We love jumpin' around to "Cherry Bomb."

33. The Sex Pistols *Never Mind the Bollocks, Here's the Sex Pistols*, 1977 (EMI). You need to have at least one of the songs on this album in your workout.

34. Siouxsie & the Banshees *The Scream*, 1978 (Geffen). When punk and Goth first combined—and it's so cool to hear a woman doing it. For those of you who only think of synthesizers and eyeliner when you hear the name Siouxsie Sioux. Worth hearing just for their spooky horror movie version of the Beatles' "Helter Skelter." Great stretching songs.

35. The Slits *Cut*, 1979 (Island). We recommend the CD reissued in 1990 on Island, which includes a cover of "I Heard It Through the Grapevine" (not to be missed).

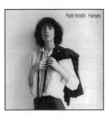

36. Patti Smith *Horses*, 1975 (Arista). Poetry in motion. One woman's vision from New Jersey, hooked up with Lenny Kaye on guitar (the guy who compiled all those great Nugget compilations) and set to music. A thread from Rimbaud and Walt Whitman continues to Patti Smith. You need to have this woman in your life. Go out and buy it.

37. Social Distortion *Mommy's Little Monster*, 1982 (13th Floor). For all the alienated and those who never fit in. This is such a great record, and the title song is our favorite.

38. SS Decontrol *The Kids Will Have Their Say*, 1982 (Dischord). This record rules. One of our favorite songs by them is "Glue" on *Get It Away*, 1983 (Xclaim!). Springer's vocals are incredible. No one we know has ever or will ever sound like him or the way he screams. Good for aggressive strength-training moves.

39. Stiff Little Fingers *Inflammable Material*, 1979 (Restless).

40. The Stranglers *Rattus Norvegicus*, 1977 (Liberty Records). Side two is the way to go. "Peaches" and "Get a Grip on Yourself" are the best songs. Don't let the weird and wordy name of the album title confuse you. This record has keyboards all over it and a groove that's superdanceable, yet totally punk.

41. Suicide *Suicide*, 1977 (Red Star). Great music. They were way before their time, and people are finally catching up. Synth punk. Listen to this record with all the lights off.

42. Swell Maps *A Trip to Marineville*, 1979 (Rough Trade). If you like Sonic Youth, Dinosaur Jr., and Pavement, see where they got some of their sound.

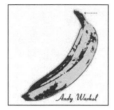

43. Television *Marquee Moon*, 1977 (Elektra/Asylum). Tom Verlaine and Richard Hell. Two punk rock heroes in this band. Great songs to leg lift to, no joke.

44. The Undertones *The Undertones*, 1979 (Sanctuary); *The Very Best of the Undertones*, 1994 (Rykodisc USA).

45. The Velvet Underground *The Velvet Underground & Nico*, 1965 (Verve). Like most great art, this record was ignored when it came out, and by the time it became a success, the group (including Lou Reed and John Cale) had broken up. An elegy to junkies and miscreants, the underbelly of America. Features the classic songs "I'm Waiting for the Man" and "Heroin."

46. The Wipers *Is This Real?* 1979 (Park Avenue). Greg Sage *is* The Wipers. You may never have heard of them because he's a guy who lives alone in the desert writing a lot of songs about alien abduction. His songs are furious and punk rock, though, with dissonant, innovative chord progressions. A little bit depressing, maybe a better cool-down song selection for your workout.

47. Wire *Pink Flag*, 1977 (Harvest); *Chairs Missing*, 1977 (Harvest); *154*, 1979 (Harvest). Totally addictive.

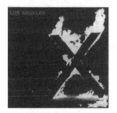

48. X *Los Angeles*, 1980 (Elektra).

49. X-Ray Spex *Germ Free Adolescents*, 1978 (Blue). Features the vocal talents of Poly Styrene, a true original.

50. XTC *Drums and Wires*, 1979 (Virgin). Easy listening, but don't knock it—chock-full of great songs to bop around to.

ACKNOWLEDGMENTS

OUR THANKS TO: Benjamin Nugent, Ami Bennitt, Kristen Driscoll, Alex Van Buren, Alex Camlin, Jud Laghi, Liz Linder, Amanda Cole, Angela Hubbard, Kris Canning, Chris Hosford, Michael Azerrad, Hank Pierce, Steven Blush, and Erica Lawrence. Thanks to everyone who posed for a photo or was interviewed for this book, especially J Mascis, Clint Conley, and Mary Timony. Thank you T.D. and Ama for teaching our classes while we worked on this book, Joseph and Nabil Sater at The Middle East Restaurant for giving us the space to make it possible, and all the cool peeps who come to class and make our Saturdays so great. Lastly, thank you to our families and to Winston and Mark for being so supportive of our crazy endeavors! Oh yeah, Evan, thanks for smashing that boombox!

Primary photography: Liz Linder, Boston.
Stylist: Amanda Cole for The Nines, Williamsburg, New York

Additional models/P.R.A. Instructors: Ama Allara of Rock City Body, Boston, and T.D. Sidell of the band The Big Digits

Additional photography: Thurston Moore (page 92) by Angela Hubbard; Dee Dee Ramone (page 43), Johnny Thunders (page xxviii) © Bob Gruen/Star File; Kim Gordon, Iggy Pop (page xxxii) by Lana Caplan; Henry Rollins (page xxxii) © Jay Hale; Calvin Johnson (page 79) by Sara S. Lee; supermarket photo (page 151) by Byrne Guarnotta.